# MAKING MANAGED HEALTH CARE WORK FOR KIDS IN FOSTER CARE:

## A Guide to Purchasing Services

*by Ellen Sittenfeld Battistelli*

*CWLA Press • Washington, DC*

CWLA Press is an imprint of the Child Welfare League of America, Inc.

© 1996 by the Child Welfare League of America, Inc.

CHILD WELFARE LEAGUE OF AMERICA, INC.
440 First Street, NW, Suite 310, Washington, DC 20001-2085
Email: books@cwla.org

CURRENT PRINTING (last digit)
10  9  8  7  6  5  4  3  2  1

Cover and text design by James Graham

Printed in the United States of America
ISBN # 0–87868–683–5

# Contents

Access to Services

Confidentiality

Benefit Packages

Specialized Medical Services

Behavioral Health Services

Immediate Eligibility

Case Management

Recordkeeping

Quality Assurance and Quality Improvement

Prior Approval

Medical Necessity

Social Necessity

State Pressure to Reduce Medicaid Costs

Contract Language

Conclusion

# Appendixes

# Acknowledgments

*Making Managed Health Care Work for Kids in Foster Care: A Guide to Purchasing Services* was written with the guidance of an exceptional advisory board, The CWLA National Advisory Committee on Managed Health Care for Children in Foster Care.

Each member of this body contributed much time, energy, and wisdom. Madelyn DeWoody Freundlich, the chair of the committee, provided the dedication, leadership, and good judgment necessary to accomplish the task. We are especially appreciative of the participation, handholding, and encouragement of Karabelle Pizzigati, Kathy Barbell, Lydia Russo, Sarah Orrick, and Mary Liepold.

The Child Welfare League of America is grateful to the Robert Wood Johnson Foundation for its generous support in this effort and its commitment to children in foster care.

# Introduction

This guide is to help purchasers of managed health care understand the complex health care and social service needs of an especially vulnerable population—children in the foster care system. In addition, this guide explains for child welfare agencies the goals and workings of managed health care.

All children are dependent on others for their care and well-being, but children in foster care are uniquely dependent upon governments and their agencies and services. Children in foster care have complex problems rooted in family, social, and environmental conditions. They often need a range of health, mental health, and developmental services to overcome the effects of abuse and neglect. Yet their care too often is inconsistent and disjointed. Many children's health needs are not assessed in a timely or appropriate way. When problems are identified, too often these children "fall through the cracks," never getting the services they need. Further complicating the situation is the fact that children may be placed at a distance from their families and may be moved abruptly and repeatedly. Many children move frequently in and out of care or from one family foster home or care facility to another.

## Who Is Responsible for Meeting the Health Care Needs of Children in Foster Care?

A major impediment to meeting the needs of children in foster care is that the responsibility for identifying their health, behavioral, and developmental problems and providing services to address them is not clearly defined. Often, public and private agencies share accountability; and many individuals have some level of responsibility for the child, including the biological parents, the foster parents, the social worker, and the primary physician.

Theoretically, multilevel responsibility should ensure the health of the child—with the state agency overseeing the entire system of care and establishing standards of care, the private foster care agency seeing that children receive medical and mental health care, and the foster parents supervising and caring for the child day to day. In practice, however, this sharing of responsibility often has had the reverse effect. Most children in foster care lack a single strong advocate who will identify their needs and make them a priority, coordinate a treatment plan, and maneuver the system. Biological parents are rarely involved in their children's health care once the children enter out-of-home placement, so in most cases they play a very limited role (Kufelt 1982; Kadushin & Martin 1988). Foster parents can play a more active role but often are not able to assure continuity of health care. Placements in foster care are temporary, children may be placed in several different foster homes in the course of care, and foster parents often are not informed about children's health problems (Halfon & Klee 1987; Schor 1989). Caseworkers, burdened by large caseloads, tend to focus on immediate crises rather than comprehensive care (Halfon & Klee 1987; Simms 1989). Physicians often struggle with incomplete medical records and no follow-up capacity.

## The Potential of Managed Health Care

Managed care is becoming a dominant factor in the organization of health care services. For many, it is a potential solution to the current fragmentation in health care. For others, it is a threat to what currently is available and means even less access and coordination of care. And for yet others, it is an unknown warranting close study.

What is clear is that managed health care is becoming the service delivery system of choice for Medicaid beneficiaries, including children, and as a result is having a growing impact on children in foster care. A number of states already have obtained freedom-of-choice waivers, which allow them to require that certain Medicaid beneficiaries enroll in health maintenance organizations (HMOs) or prepaid health plans (PHPs). Waivers have allowed many states to mandate managed care for Medicaid beneficiaries as part of research and demonstration programs. Managed care is extending itself from the traditional health care context into mental health and social services. Ideally, this will result in better utilization and coordination of services, but it will also involve blending a variety of governmental funding streams and cost shifting between systems of care.

As the environment has evolved to managed care, questions and concerns have arisen about the impact the change will have on the health care of children in foster care. Ideally, a managed care system could accommodate the specific needs of children in foster care and could remedy the fragmentation of the current system. Managed care's emphasis on prevention, continuous coordinated care, and extensive recordkeeping could result in greater accountability.

Little attention, however, is being given to the potentially negative impacts of managed care on children in foster care. While some experts have focused on national health care reform and Medicaid as they relate to children in foster care, there has been no concerted effort to specifically analyze managed care's focus on reducing service utilization with regard to the service needs of children and young people in foster care.

This guide has been developed out of a recognition that health care delivery and financing for this group of youngsters must be addressed in light of the realities of managed care and that managed care must be examined in light of how it can be made to work effectively for children in foster care.

Child welfare agencies have lacked specific guidelines and information to help them assess and develop health care policies and programs that meet the specific needs of children in foster care. This guide is designed to fill that gap.

## Goals of This Guide

The guide has two main objectives:

- to help the designers and purchasers of managed health care plans and managed care organizations understand the child welfare system and the children it serves and design effective health care programs as they expand their Medicaid managed care programs to children and young people with special health care needs; and

- to help child welfare agencies understand the managed care environment and become more effective at working with Medicaid agencies and managed care companies and promoting the health of children.

To achieve these objectives, this guide provides

- an explanation of how the Medicaid, managed care, and foster care systems operate;

- an overview of the special health, mental health, developmental, and rehabilitative needs of children in foster care;

- a checklist of health care services and supportive services that contracts with managed care organizations must include and procedures to ensure that managed care organizations meet these needs appropriately;

- an examination of the state's legal responsibilities for the health of children in foster care;

- an outline of steps that child welfare service providers and advocates must take to ensure that managed care approaches meet children's needs;

- a list of questions for the child welfare worker to ask about services available from the state's plan; and

- suggestions on how to expand eligibility for children's services (including greater access to prevention and early intervention services), increase flexibility in service design and delivery, identify and overcome potential barriers to services (such as inappropriate "medical necessity" criteria) and ensure increased accountability and greater emphasis on outcomes.

It is hoped that this guide, along with its companion volume, *A Guide to Managed Care for Foster Parents and Caregivers*, will bridge the gap between two systems that share responsibility for meeting the broad and complex needs of children and young people in foster care: the child welfare system and managed care service delivery and financing systems.

Ultimately, the goal is to provide children in foster care with appropriate, accessible, and high-quality services that will help them develop physically, emotionally, and intellectually. Progress toward this goal will pay off for years to come, not only for the individual child but for society as a whole.

## References

Halfon, N., & Klee, L. (1987, August). Health services for California's foster children: Current practices and policy recommendations. *Pediatrics 80* (2), 183–191.

Kadushin, A., & Martin, J. A. (1988). *Child Welfare Services* (4th ed.). New York: Macmillan.

Schor, E.L. (1989, January). Foster care. *Pediatrics in Review 10* (7), 209–216.

Simms, M.D. (1989). The foster care clinic: A community program to identify treatment needs of children in foster care. *Journal of Developmental and Behavioral Pediatrics 10,* 121–128.

# Chapter One

# Foster Children and Health Care

To address the health care needs of children in foster care most effectively, it is necessary to understand the foster care* system itself: what it is, who it serves, and which individuals and organizations are responsible for providing care. This chapter describes the foster care system, the children who are in the system, and their special health care needs.

## What Is Foster Care?

The removal of a child from his or her parents is a drastic act undertaken only when there is imminent danger to the child's life and health, or when other measures to alleviate risk have failed or can not provide sufficient protection. When the child is subject to such imminent harm, child welfare agencies are authorized to intervene and, with the approval of the court, place the child in foster care. Foster care provides children with care and nurturing away from their parents and in the home of an agency-approved family, in a group home, or in a residential setting for a limited period of time. It is hoped that while the child is in foster care, the biological parents, with the help of the child welfare system, will learn to manage or resolve their personal and social problems so they can again take care of their child.

---

\*    CWLA publications generally use *out-of-home care* as the inclusive term, then distinguish between family foster care and group residential care. In this volume, however, the term *foster care* is used to cover both categories of care, and *foster children* denotes all children in out-of-home care.

Every state administers child welfare programs. When children are in foster care, the state child welfare agency is obligated to provide a range of services to the child, including health care, and to the parents to help them overcome the problems that led to the removal of the child from their custody. Services for parents often include counseling, parenting education, and linkages with income assistance and housing.

The goal of child welfare agencies is to protect children from abuse and neglect and to support and preserve families. Agencies investigate reports of child abuse and neglect; work with families with problems and, when necessary, seek court approval to remove children from their parents' custody; provide foster care for children who must be separated from their parents; and, whenever possible, reunite children safely and permanently with their biological families.

Over the last several years, foster care has become a system under siege. The population of children in care has skyrocketed, the needs of these children have become increasingly complex, children are remaining in care for extended periods of time, and many children who have been returned to their families are reentering the system. At the same time, resources to support the system have remained level or have declined, leading to what virtually all observers would describe as an overburdened, underfunded system. As caseloads have grown, staff turnover has escalated, reports of children being maltreated and neglected while in foster care have reached the public, and there has been increasing concern about the health and well-being of children in care.

## Who Are the Children in Foster Care, and How Do They Enter the System?

Three decades ago, children were most often placed in foster care as a result of a parent's physical or mental illness or death or the financial inability of the family to care for them. In the 1970s, neglect and abuse became the more frequent precipitating causes for children entering care.

The ability of parents to care for their children can be weakened seriously by poverty, single and too-early parenthood, mental illness,

## Figure 1. Types of Maltreatment

In the 1994 cases of substantiated abuse and neglect, of the children involved,

- 53% were neglected,

- 26% were physically abused,

- 14% were sexually abused,

- 5% were emotionally abused,

- 3% were medically neglected, and

- 15% were classified as suffering from another form of abuse.

**Source:** U.S. Department of Health and Human Services, National Center on Child Abuse and Neglect. (1996). *Child Maltreatment 1994: Reports from the States to the National Center on Child Abuse and Neglect.* Washington, DC: U.S. Government Printing Office.

homelessness, and joblessness. In the 1980s, with the advent of crack cocaine, parental drug involvement became a major reason for the increased number of children entering foster care. These dynamics remain in the 1990s, and new populations—including children who are HIV positive and children who have lost their parents to AIDS—are entering foster care. Children and parents continue to be separated as a result of homelessness, which also delays family reunification once children enter foster care [Barbell 1995]. In 1988, homelessness was a factor in over 40% of placements into foster care in New Jersey, and the sole precipitating cause in 18% [Ooms 1990].

In 1994, nearly three million children in the United States were reported physically, emotionally, or sexually abused or neglected [HHS 1996]. From 1976 to 1993, the rate of child abuse and neglect reporting increased 331% [HHS 1995]. For 37% of the investigated reports, abuse and neglect were either substantiated or indicated [HHS 1996]. Of the children whose reports were substantiated in 1994, 53% were neglected, 26% were physically abused, 14% were sexually abused, 5% were emotionally abused, 3% were medically neglected, and 15% were classified as suffering from another form of abuse. Child protective service agencies in 35 states reported that 126,117 maltreated children (15% of those reported) were removed from their homes in 1994 [HHS 1996].

In 1993, 449,000 children and youths were in foster care in the United States. This represents a 61% increase from 1984, when the total was 246,000 children [Tatara 1994]. Four factors have contributed to the dramatic increases in the numbers of children in foster care:

- an increase in the number of reports of child abuse and neglect,

- increasing rates of reentry into foster care,

- increasing length of time that children spend in care, and

- the impact of other service systems, such as mental health and the courts, on the number of children and young people whom the foster care system serves. [Barbell 1995]

Substance abuse, in particular, has had a significant impact on children, young people, and families, and has become an important precipitating factor in the placement of children in foster care [CWLA 1992]. The abuse of crack cocaine, alcohol, and other dangerous drugs has contributed to the soaring incidence of child abuse, neglect, and abandonment reported in recent years. A 1989 Boston study concluded that parental alcohol or drug abuse was a factor in 89% of all known child abuse or neglect involving children under age one [Hershowitz et al. 1989].

According to a 1994 report by the U.S. General Accounting Office (GAO), alcohol and drug abuse are factors in the placement of more than 75% of the children who enter care [GAO 1994]. Drug abuse is also related to the growing number of boarder babies—infants who remain in hospitals simply because they have nowhere else to go. Fully 85% of the boarder babies identified in a 1991 CWLA survey of 72 hospitals in 12 cities had been exposed to alcohol or other drugs prenatally [CWLA 1992, June]. A 1993 report from the Children's Bureau, U.S. Department of Health and Human

Services (HHS), counted 22,000 boarder babies and abandoned infants in the United States in 1991. Over three-fourths of these children were found to be drug exposed [HHS 1993].

Children in foster care come from all racial and ethnic groups, all income levels, and all types of families and communities. Often, they come from poor, minority, and single-parent families. Frequently, family members suffer from mental health problems, substance abuse, homelessness, or physical disability. Their neighborhoods are impoverished urban areas with high rates of crime, violence, and drug abuse. Many parents of children in foster care were themselves abused and neglected.

In 1990, 61% of the children in foster care were children of color—African American, Native American, or Latino [Tatara 1993]. Because of this, the child welfare system has had to become more responsive to cultural and ethnic diversity in recent years. Agencies must consider the child's and family's sociocultural environment in order to understand their problems and their motivations to change.

Children coming into the child welfare system today are significantly different from the children of the 1980s, "with a growing number of seriously handicapped infants at one end of the spectrum, and a preponderance of emotionally disabled teenagers at the other end" [APWA 1990]. As a group:

*Today, children in foster care are young.*

- Infants and young children with medical complications and physical and mental limitations constitute the fastest-growing group of children in need of foster care. [House of Representatives 1989]. Infants constitute nearly 25% of all entries into foster care [Goerge et al. 1994].

*Today, children in foster care have serious disabilities.*

- Children are entering out-of-home care at younger ages; with more serious and complex problems; and suffering from physical, sexual, or emotional abuse, alcohol or drug exposure, HIV infection, poverty, and homelessness [Halfon et al. 1993].

*Today, a significant number of children are in foster care because of AIDS.*

- An estimated 80,000 healthy children will be orphaned by AIDS before the year 2000, with approximately one-third of that number expected to enter the child welfare system [Taylor et al. 1993].

*Today, children who previously were served by the mental health and the juvenile justice systems are entering foster care.*

- Policies mandating deinstitutionalization of children with mental health problems and decriminalization of status offenders— that is, young people charged with running away, ungovernability, truancy, or liquor-law violations—have increased the number of emotionally disturbed, mentally ill, developmentally disabled, and delinquent children in foster care [National Commission on Children 1991; NFPA 1994; Barbell 1995]. Between 1984 and 1990, the number of children who entered foster care after committing status and delinquent offenses increased 52% [Tatara 1993].

*Today, significant numbers of drug-exposed infants are entering foster care.*

- At the same time, a growing population of infants and very young children born to or being raised by parents who abuse drugs are entering foster care. Many of these children were exposed to drugs in utero and born to mothers who did not receive appropriate prenatal care. As a result, many have physical, psychological, and developmental disabilities. Some are at risk for developing AIDS because their mothers are infected with HIV.

## Who Is Responsible for Children in Foster Care?

Children in foster care are truly and legally the children of our society. Removing children from the custody of their parents is an extreme act with serious consequences for the children, the families, and society.

## Figure 2. Children in the Child Welfare System Today

- Foster children are young.

- Foster children have serious disabilities.

- A significant number of children are in foster care because of AIDS.

- Children who previously would have been served by the mental health system are now in foster care.

- Children who otherwise would have entered the juvenile justice system are now served by the foster care system.

- Significant numbers of drug-exposed infants are in foster care.

## Governments

When the state, on behalf of the community, determines that the separation of a child from parents is in that child's best interests because of an imminent risk of serious harm, it must ensure that all basic needs, including physical and emotional care, are properly provided for in an improved environment [CWLA 1989]. The responsibility for providing care and services is shared by federal, state, and county governments. HSS has oversight of federally mandated safeguards for children in foster care, and state and county governments have the responsibility for implementing and monitoring foster care programs.

## Courts

The court is the only authority that may limit or terminate parental rights and transfer custody of a child to a designated individual or agency. When a court places a child in foster care, it can direct a plan for the child's care and treatment, including health care.

## Child Welfare Agencies

Child welfare agencies are charged with protecting children, rebuilding families, or finding permanent families for children through adoption, and for ensuring the health and well-being of children in their care. Child welfare agencies, in effect, take on parental responsibilities for children in foster care—legally, ethically, and morally. They may do this by arranging for family foster care or by providing on-site residential care and services. The escalating number of children in out-of-home care, their heightened vulnerability and need for services, and inadequate resources overwhelm many public child welfare systems.

## Social Workers

A child welfare agency social worker is responsible for overseeing a plan that ensures protection and care of the child, for developing a permanency plan for the child, for placing a child with an agency-approved foster family, and for working with the foster family to see that the child's physical, mental health, developmental, social, and educational needs are met. This responsibility includes providing the resources to meet the range of the child's needs and providing case management services to ensure access to appropriate services. Social workers must elicit necessary health-related information from the parents or guardians, previous health care providers, and case records.

## Foster Families

Foster families are charged with the daily protection, care, and nurturing of children who must live away from their parents for a limited period of time. The foster family and social workers must act as partners in meeting the ongoing health, emotional, developmental, educational, and social needs of the child in care.

As the number of American children needing out-of-home care increased, between 1985 and 1994 the number of foster family providers steadily declined from 147,000 to 125,000 [National Foster Parent Association 1994]. This decline is due to a number of factors, including social and economic changes in our societ, but it is also due to increased demands on foster families. Foster parents today are asked to care for children with very complex and special medical, developmental, and behavioral needs [Barbell 1995].

## Figure 3. A Snapshot of Children in Foster Care, 1990

- 50% were placed for protective-service reasons (abuse or neglect that places the child at imminent risk of serious harm).

- 21% were placed because of parental condition or absence (illness, financial hardship, disability, or death).

- 11% were placed because the child committed status or delinquent offenses.

- 2% were placed because of the child's disability.

- 1% were placed because parental rights had been relinquished.

- 13% were placed for state-defined reasons, including a parent-child relationship problem or family interaction problem, an adoption or subsidized adoption plan, or deinstitutionalization.

**Source:** Tatara, T. (1993, October). *Characteristics of children in substitute and adoptive care.* Washington, DC: American Public Welfare Association, Voluntary Cooperative Information System.

Historically, foster parents have been reimbursed at very low rates for the care they provide. They are expected to subsidize the child welfare system through their time and out–of–pocket expenses for services such as child day care [Barbell 1995]. Foster parenting is essentially a volunteer program that depends on the good intentions and natural abilities of generous lay people. In too many cases, foster parents receive inadequate training and support from agency social workers [Barbell 1995].

## Physicians

Given the substantial health problems of children in foster care, the demands upon the primary health care provider are extensive and time consuming. The provider must be aware of the entirety of the child's health and social needs and be able to ensure that the child receives the comprehensive, continuous, and accessible care required. Few physicians have extensive experience in caring for large numbers of children in foster care.

Because of low reimbursement rates, the number of physicians participating in Medicaid dropped between 1978 and 1989 [Yudkowsk et al. 1990].

## What Happens to Children in Foster Care?

More than 73% of the children in out-of-home care are placed in family foster homes, including specialized and therapeutic homes [Tatara 1993]. The remainder are in child care institutions, emergency shelters, or group homes. A very few are in juvenile justice facilities and mental health institutions.

A primary goal of child welfare is reuniting children and families. About 90% of children who enter foster care will be reunited with their parents eventually. Even when children are prepared for independent living, 60% ultimately return to live with their families [DeWoody et al. 1993].

Nearly two-thirds of the children who left foster care in FY 1990 either were reunited with their families or placed with the other parent, a relative, or a caregiver. Another 6.5% were emancipated or reached the age of majority, whereas 7.7% were adopted. Some 15.7% of children left care for other reasons, including running away, incarceration, marriage, death, discharge to another public agency, or the establishment of legal guardianship [Tatara 1993].

Reunification does not always work. Thirty percent of the children who were reunited with families after entering foster care in 1983 reentered foster care by the end of 1993 [Goerge et al. 1994; Barbell 1996]. If children are not discharged within a short time after the initial placement in foster care, they are likely to remain in care for long periods of time [Merkel-Holguin 1993]. The length of time a child is likely to remain in care varies widely between states and among the different subgroups within each state: urban-rural, race, ethnicity, and age [Goerge et al. 1994].

## Figure 4. Reuniting Foster Children and Their Families

- An estimated 90% of children who enter foster care will be reunited with their families.

- Some 60% of youths being prepared to live independently ultimately return to live with their families.

- Nearly two-thirds of the children who left foster care in FY 1990 either were reunited with their families or placed with the other parent, a relative, or another caregiver.

- Of children who were reunited with their families after entering foster care in 1983, 30% had reentered foster care by the end of 1993.

# What Are the Special Health Needs of Children in Foster Care?

Most children enter foster care in a poor state of health [Simms & Halfon 1994], and most enter care with developmental, behavioral, and emotional disturbances [Simms & Halfon 1994; Schor 1982; Moffatt et al. 1985; Hochstadt et al. 1987; Kadushin & Martin 1988; Simms 1989; and Halfon 1992a]. Even when compared with other children of the same socioeconomic background, children in foster care suffer much higher rates of serious emotional and behavioral problems, chronic physical disabilities, birth defects, developmental delays, and poor school achievement [American Academy of Pediatrics 1994].

When children enter care, they come with conditions directly or indirectly resulting from parental neglect or abuse. Many of these children started their lives at low birthweights, prenatally exposed to illegal drugs or alcohol, or exposed to HIV–AIDS and other diseases [Schor 1988]. Neglect and abuse may occur when a family's emotional and financial resources are taxed by the demands of a disabled child [Simms 1996].

The extent of the health care problems that face abused and neglected children is truly alarming [Schor 1982; Hochstadt et al. 1987; Simms 1989; Halfon 1992a]. In a 1995 GAO study, 62% of young children in foster care had been subject to prenatal drug exposure. This places them at risk for serious health problems in infancy and throughout their lives. An increasing number of infants who enter care have multiple health and developmental needs. Children in foster care and their families often have lacked adequate health care. Children often are behind in their immunizations or have undiagnosed health problems and developmental delays.

Adolescents in foster care are at higher than normal risk for abuse of alcohol or drugs and for sexual activity that can lead to contracting and transmitting HIV infection and to becoming teen parents. They often have learning disabilities, school failures, chronic illnesses, and untreated psychological problems. Further, the troubled parents who come to the attention of the child welfare system seldom have received the physical care, mental health services, or substance abuse treatment they need.

*Chronic medical problems* affect 30% to 40% of children in the child welfare system. These problems include delayed growth and development; HIV infection; neurological disabilities; malnutrition; asthma; anemia; poor vision; ear infections; hearing problems; tooth decay; failure to thrive; musculoskeletal deformities; and dermatologic, allergic, and orthodontic problems [Schor 1988; Simms & Halfon 1994]. Short stature is two to three times as common in children in foster care as in the general population [Schor 1988; Simms 1989; Halfon et al. 1995]. Sexually transmitted diseases are seen more commonly in this group than in other children of similar ages [Flaherty & Weiss 1990]. Often, these chronic recurrent conditions have been untreated or only partially treated [Schor 1988].

*Mental health problems,* especially depression, are particularly widespread among children in foster care. Some experts believe that emotional problems are almost universal in children in foster care [Schor 1988]. The prevalence of mental health and developmental problems has been estimated at 12% to 15% in the general child population and 35% to 85% in the foster care population [Halfon et al. 1992a; Simms & Halfon 1994 citing Schor 1982; Moffatt et al.

1985; Hochstadt et al. 1987; Simms 1989]. These problems include conduct disorders, depression, difficulties in school, and impaired social relationships [Barbell 1996]. Halfon et al. [1992a] found that conduct, adjustment, anxiety, and emotional disorders represented 75% of all diagnoses of children in foster care.

One estimate is that over one-third of children in foster care have moderate to severe emotional problems and another third have evident, although less severe, disabilities [Schor 1988]. It is believed that at least 20% of these children have emotional problems serious enough to warrant referral for ongoing psychotherapy.

Research has shown that children who suffer maltreatment experience a wide range of behavioral and emotional problems, including low self-esteem, aggression, depression, cognitive impairment, communication difficulties, conduct disorders, and delinquency [Halfon et al. 1992a]. The frequency and severity of emotional problems among children in foster care seem to be strongly related to their history of deprivation, neglect, and abuse and to the lack of security and permanence in their lives [Schor 1988].

*Developmental disabilities* affect a high proportion of children who are abused or neglected. Many of the children coming into care are medically fragile and/or physically handicapped [Barbell 1995]. Between 1984 and 1990, there was a 12% increase in the number of children who entered foster care because their own disabilities made it difficult for their parents to care for them [Tatara 1993]. A nationwide study revealed that approximately 20% of children in out-of-home care have developmental disabilities—mental retardation, cerebral palsy, and learning disabilities, as well as speech, hearing, and sight impairments. The rate is twice as high for preschool children in foster care. This high rate of developmental disabilities appears to contribute to subsequent educational failures [Simms & Halfon 1994].

## Why Is Comprehensive Health Care Important?

Because children in foster care are "sicker than homeless children and children living in the poorest sections of inner cities" [GAO 1995], they require a disproportionate amount of health care services, compared with other children who receive Medicaid [Halfon et al. 1992a and 1992b.] At the same time, the care they usually do receive is neither coordinated nor comprehensive.

Children usually enter care having had limited contact with the health care system. The early lack of comprehensive health care often is exacerbated by family disorganization and the abuse and neglect they have experienced. The separation from their families inherent in foster care placement also can seriously impact the mental health status of these children [Schor 1988; Halfon et al. 1992b]. Each phase of foster care placement may bring new traumas and disruptions to already vulnerable children [Molin 1988; Schor 1989; Halfon et al. 1992a].

In general, children in foster care get too little health care—and often the wrong kind. Few children enter care with a complete health history [Klee & Halfon 1987]. Often, their health records are scattered and incomplete. Immunization records are usually lacking [Klee & Halfon 1987]. Children may fall through the cracks of a bureaucracy in which caseworkers and foster parents change so often that identified problems are not followed up on and ongoing care is disrupted [Simms & Halfon 1994; Schor 1988]. Because there is little continuity in caregiving, and recordkeeping often is inadequate and incomplete, they may have to start over in their medical and mental health treatments.

The significant need of children in foster care for higher-end health care services is demonstrated by statistics on medical utilization by children in foster care:

- Children in foster care use more health care services than other children covered by Medicaid. The average cost per child is higher than for other Medicaid children, and this differential utilization increases with age [Halfon et al. 1992a].

- AFDC children in foster care cost six times more per capita in health care spending than AFDC children not in foster care— $3,075 per year verses $543 per year [Takayama 1994].

The benefits of comprehensive care are well documented. Research shows that when children in foster care receive appropriate care, they show significant improvement in their physical, emotional, and intellectual development [Fanshel & Shinn 1978; White & Benedict 1986; Simms & Halfon 1994]. "Preventive care, early treatment of acute illnesses, and amelioration of chronic illnesses early in life may prevent more costly health problems later" [Perkins & Rivera 1995, citing the National Governors' Association 1991]. Conversely, the failure to provide necessary services heightens the risk of problems becoming more serious. Conditions left untreated can influence functioning into adulthood. Whether children are in or out of foster care, dollars spent on prevention and early intervention avert the need for more expensive and intensive services later.

Placement in foster care is an opportunity to address the physical and emotional health care needs of the children who are in greatest need of such services. In fact, federal law requires that the case plan for a child in foster care include the child's health records, and that these records be reviewed and updated. Foster care is a service that can bring together social work and health care expertise and connect children with services to which they previously had little or no access. It should be—and can be—an ideal environment for marshaling the resources that vulnerable children need. Doing so can shorten the length of placement in foster care [Simms & Halfon 1994; Horwitz, et al. 1994]. Logically, this decreases the costs to the system and increases the chances of successful reunification or adoption.

The challenge comes in guaranteeing children in foster care both the preventive and primary care all children need and the specialized services they particularly need. Children in foster care have complex problems and require a broad range of physical, mental health, and supplemental services to overcome the effects of abuse and neglect. These children have unique needs—physical, emotional, and social—that result from the interplay of their histoies, their placement in out-of-home care, and the stress and instability of their situations [Klee & Halfon 1987]. The challenges involved in ensuring continuous comprehensive health coverage for these children may be enormous, but they can be met through a commitment to improving these children's health and well-being, thoughtful planning, and provision of accessible services.

# References

American Academy of Pediatrics (AAP), Committee on Early Childhood, Adoption, and Dependent Care. (1994, February). Health care of children in foster care. *Pediatrics 93* (2), 1–4.

American Public Welfare Association (APWA). (1990). *A commitment to change: Report of the National Commission on Child Welfare and Family Preservation.* Washington, DC: Author.

Barbell, K. (1995). *Foster care today: A briefing paper.* Washington, DC: Child Welfare League of America.

Barbell, K. (1996, March). *Foster Care F.Y.I.* #1 Washington, DC: Child Welfare League of America.

Child Welfare League of America (CWLA). (1989). *Standards for service for abused or neglected children and their families.* Washington DC: Author.

Child Welfare League of America (CWLA), North American Commission on Chemical Dependency and Child Welfare. (1992). *Children at the front: A different view of the war on alcohol and drugs.* Washington, DC:.

Child Welfare League of America (CWLA) and the National Association of Public Hospitals. (1992, June). *The youngest of the homeless II: A survey of boarder babies in selected hospitals in the United States.* Washington, DC: Author.

DeWoody, M., Ceja, K., & Sylvester, M. (1993). *Independent living services for youths in out-of-home care.* Washington, DC: Child Welfare League of America.

Fanshell, D., & Shinn, E.G. (1978). *Children in foster care: A longitudinal investigation.* New York: Columbia University Press.

Flaherty, E.G., & Weiss, H. (1990, March). Medical evaluation of abused and neglected children. *American Journal of Diseases of Children 144,* 330–334.

Goerge, R.M., Wulczyn, F.H., & Harden, A.W. (1994). *Foster care dynamics 1983–1992: A report from the multistate foster care data archive.* Chicago: Chapin Hall Center for Children at the University of Chicago.

Halfon, N., Berkowitz, G., & Klee, L. (1992a). Children in foster care in California: An examination of Medicaid reimbursed health services utilization. *Pediatrics 89,* 1230–1237.

Halfon, N., Berkowitz, G., & Klee, L. (1992b). Mental health service utilization by children in foster care in California. *Pediatrics 89,* 1238–1244.

Halfon, N., Berkowitz, G., & Klee, L. (1993). Development of an integrated case management program for vulnerable children. *Child Welfare LXXII* (4), 379–396.

Halfon, N., Mendonca, A., & Berkowitz, G. (1995, April). Health status of children in foster care. *ARCH Pediatric Adolescent Medicine 149,* 386–392.

Hershowitz, J., Seck, M., & Fogg, C. (1989, June). *Substance abuse and family violence.* Boston: Massachusetts Department of Social Services.

Hochstadt, N., Jaudes, P., Zimo, D., & Schachter, J. (1987). The medical and psychosocial needs of children entering foster care. *Child Abuse and Neglect 11,* 3–62.

Horwitz, S.M., Simms, M., & Farrington, R.M. (1994, April). Impact of developmental problems on young children's exits from foster care. *Journal of Developmental and Behavioral Pediatrics 15* (2), 105–110.

Kadushin, A., & Martin, J. A. (1988). *Child welfare services* (4th ed.). New York: Macmillan.

Klee, L., & Halfon, N. (1987). Mental health care for foster children in California. *Child Abuse and Neglect 11*, 63–74.

Merkel-Holguin, L. (1993). *The child welfare stat book 1993*. Washington, DC: Child Welfare League of America.

Moffatt, M.E.K., Peddie, M., Stulginskas, J., et al. (1985). Health care delivery to foster children: A study. *Health and Social Work 10*, 129–137.

Molin, R. (1988). Treatment of children in foster care: Issues of collaboration. *Child Abuse and Neglect 12*, 241–249.

National Commission on Children. (1991). *Beyond rhetoric: A new American agenda for children and families*. Washington, DC: Author.

National Foster Parent Association, Inc. (1994, May). A survey of the states 1994. A report at the 1994 NFPA national conference.

Ooms, T. (1990). *The crisis in foster care: New directions for the 1990s*. Washington, DC: Family Impact Seminars. (Background briefing report and meeting highlights).

Perkins, J., & Rivera, L. (1995, July). *Medicaid managed care: 20 questions to ask your state*. San Francisco: National Health Law Program.

Schor, E.L. (1982, May). The foster care system and the health status of foster children. *Pediatrics 69* (5), 521–528.

Schor, E.L. (1988, December). Foster care. *The Pediatric Clinics of North America 35* (6), 1241–1252.

Schor, E.L. (1989, January). Foster care. *Pediatrics in Review 10* (7), 209–216.

Simms, M.D. (1989). The foster care clinic: A community program to identify treatment needs of children in foster care. *Journal of Developmental and Behavioral Pediatrics 10*, 121–128.

Simms, M.D. (1996, June). *Health issues of children in the foster care system*. Handout accompanying presentation at Vail, CO.

Simms, M.D., & Halfon, N. (1994, September–October). The health care needs of children in foster care: A research agenda. *Child Welfare LXXIII*(5), 505–524.

Takayama, J. (1994). Children in foster care in the state of Washington: Health care utilization and expenditures. *Journal of the American Medical Association 271* (23).

Tatara, T. (1993, October). *Characteristics of children in substitute and adoptive care*. Washington, DC: American Public Welfare Association, Voluntary Cooperative Information System.

Tatara, T. (1994, October). *Characteristics of children in substitute and adoptive care*. Washington, DC: American Public Welfare Association, Voluntary Cooperative Information System.

Taylor-Brown, S., Wilcyzinski, C., Moore, E., & Cohen, F. (1992). Perinatal AIDS: Permanency planning for the African American community. Journal of Multicultural Social Work 2 (3), 85–100.

U.S. Department of Health and Human Services (HHS), Administration for Children and Families, Children's Bureau. (1993, August). *Report to Congress: National estimates on the number of boarder babies, the cost of their care, and the number of abandoned infants*. Washington, DC: Government Printing Office.

U.S. Department of Health and Human Services (HHS), National Center on Child Abuse and Neglect. (1995). *Child maltreatment 1993: Reports from the states to the National Center on Child Abuse and Neglect.* Washington, DC: Government Printing Office.

U.S. Department of Health and Human Services, National Center on Child Abuse and Neglect. (1996). *Child maltreatment 1994: Reports from the states to the National Center on Child Abuse and Neglect.* Washington, DC: Government Printing Office.

U.S. General Accounting Office (GAO). (1994, April). Foster care: Parental drug abuse has alarming impact on young children. Washington, DC: Author (GAO/HEHS-94-89).

U.S. General Accounting Office (GAO). (1995, May). Foster care: Health needs of many young children are unknown and unmet. Washington, DC: Author (GAO/HEHS-95-114).

U.S. House of Representatives, Select Committee on Children, Youth, and Families. (1989, November). *No place to call home: Discarded children in America.* Washington, DC: Government Printing Office.

White, R., & Benedict, M. (1986, April). Health status and utilization patterns of children in foster care: Executive summary (Monograph).

Yudkowsky, B.K., Cartland, J.D.C., & Flint, S.S. (1990). Pediatrician participation in Medicaid: 1978 to 1989. *Pediatrics 85,* 567–577.

# Chapter Two

## Medicaid and Managed Care

Health care in the United States is in the throes of staggering change. Rapidly increasing health care costs and rising numbers of people without insurance have prompted a national focus on health care. In its first two years, the Clinton Administration dedicated an unprecedented amount of time to reforming the nation's health care system and assuring health care to all Americans. The effort failed. In 1995 and 1996, the 104th Congress, under the rein of newly empowered Republican leadership, targeted federal health care programs—specifically Medicare and Medicaid—for programmatic change and massive cuts in projected spending. The result was legislative gridlock.

But while the federal government stumbles in its effort to reshape the health care system, the marketplace is reshaping itself. Moved by escalating costs and inefficient operations, insurance companies and fiscal intermediaries are creating managed care systems. Hospitals and medical practices are merging, aligning, downsizing, or disappearing. Corporations, looking to control spending on employee health care benefits, steer their employees to prepaid health plans and other managed care arrangements. State governments, overwhelmed by growing Medicaid costs, are enrolling their low-income populations in managed care.

There are many questions about the impact of these new health care financing and delivery arrangements on patients, providers, and the parties who pay for services. Especially unclear is the significance of these changes for children in foster care, an underserved, high-risk population with unusually complicated health and mental health needs. This chapter discusses what Medicaid, managed health care, and Medicaid managed care mean for children in foster care.

## Medicaid

Medicaid, Title XIX of the Social Security Act, is a program financed by each state, in partnership with the federal government, that purchases medical care services for low-income children, families, and the elderly. It is governed by a maze of federal and state laws, regulations, and guidelines. Because Medicaid is complex and has become costly to operate, governors in virtually every state are seeking to restructure the program.

Medicaid is a means-tested program with strict eligibility rules that vary from state to state. State Medicaid agencies, within broad federal mandates, determine what types of benefits will be provided, which professionals may provide the services, and what reimbursement rates will be paid for services. All children in foster care in the United States are categorically eligible for Medicaid if they receive support in foster care under the federal Adoption Assistance and Child Welfare Act, Title IV-E of the Social Security Act. Children may receive this federal foster care assistance if their biological families received or were eligible to receive Aid to Families with Dependent Children (AFDC) before the children's placement. Many states have elected to cover under Medicaid other children in foster care who are not Title IV-E eligible, through eligibility criteria such as the Ribicoff provision of the Medicaid statute (Section 1905a(i) of the Social Security Act).* As a result, Medicaid has become the primary health care payor for children in foster care.

### Early Periodic Screening, Diagnosis, and Treatment

States must meet certain federal requirements in designing their Medicaid programs. For example, they must offer the Early Periodic Screening, Diagnosis, and Treatment Program (EPSDT) to all Medicaid-eligible children. Added to the Medicaid program in 1967, and substantially revised in 1989, EPSDT offers a broad array of health care screening and treatment services for eligible children. Despite the federal mandate, states vary dramatically in their deliv-

---

\*       The Ribicoff provision authorizes the coverage of children up to age 21 who are not within the mandated Medicaid categories of recipients whom a state must cover. A state may cover all children in this category, or it may create reasonable categories of children, such as children in privately subsidized foster care and children in certain institutional settings.

ery of EPSDT services. Nonetheless, EPSDT is a useful model for the provision of preventive and primary care and remedial health services for children.

Under EPSDT, health care screenings are scheduled at established intervals. These must include assessments of the child's medical, developmental, vision, hearing, dental, and mental health; must include a comprehensive physical examination; must include appropriate immunizations and indicated laboratory tests; and can provide health education.

When a screening identifies a physical or mental defect, illness, or condition, EPSDT requires states to provide all the additional diagnostic, treatment, and follow-up services listed in Medicaid law that are medically necessary to remedy the condition. Consequently, although a state may not ordinarily provide the service under its Medicaid plan, it becomes a mandated service for a particular child when the EPSDT screen identifies a defect, illness, or condition for which the service is required. Federal law stipulates that the amount, scope, and duration of EPSDT services must be sufficient to reasonably achieve the purposes for which those services are provided. This mandate was designed to ensure that treatment and follow-up services are adequate to correct or remedy the child's problems.

## The Downside

The promises of Medicaid, and of the EPSDT program in particular, never have been fully realized. Although states are required to provide certain services, these services never have reached all those who need them. When services are covered under Medicaid, major obstacles may prevent their actual delivery. An especially significant problem is that health care providers have been reluctant to participate in the program. Many providers—family physicians, pediatricians, dentists, and even hospitals—refuse to accept Medicaid patients because they believe Medicaid payments are too low.

## Managed Health Care

Traditionally, health care in the United States has been a system of indemnity health insurance and fee-for-service medicine. In this system, patients choose their providers. The provider performs the services deemed necessary, and the insurance company pays some predetermined percentage of the bill—often 80%. Fee-for-service links health care decisions to payment for services and—many believe—offers health care providers economic incentives to provide too many services, resulting in waste and unnecessary care.

Managed care responds to this concern by offering a more tightly organized system than the traditional one. Managed care organizations control health care choices, services, and costs. A key component of managed care is the integration of financing and delivery of health care services. Managed care organizations (MCOs) not only pay for services but also propose and enforce limits on who receives care, who can provide the care, what care they receive, and for how long. MCOs contain the cost of health care by closely monitoring how health care providers treat specific illnesses and conditions, curbing tests, limiting referrals to specialists, and requiring preauthorization for expensive treatment.

In traditional fee-for-service arrangements, payors such as insurance companies bear the risk: If the cost of services exceeds the premiums collected, the insurance company loses money. Managed care companies use a variety of payment strategies that tend to shift the financial risk to the provider and/or control the costs of providing services. The two major types of managed care are risk-based contracting and non–risk-based primary care case management (PCCM). Under risk-based managed care, Medicaid, for example, contracts with a managed care organization to provide or arrange to provide an agreed-upon set of services for an established fee. The MCO may or may not then pass some risk to the providers in its network. Non–risk-based PCCM is a system of assigning responsibility for the care of a Medicaid beneficiary to a specific primary care provider. The provider receives an administrative fee for each patient each month, in addition to a fee for service, and is responsible for overseeing the patient's health care and access to services.

The three most common reimbursement mechanisms under managed care are

- *Capitation:* A method that pays a fixed amount per patient, regardless of the number or type of services the patient requires. Rather than charging for each service, MCOs receive a preset fee to meet an agreed-upon set of health care needs. If the MCO's costs in providing services exceed the prepaid fees, the MCO loses money. If costs are less than fees, the MCO makes a profit.

- *Fee Schedules:* A method that pays for services according to a pre-set fee for each service.

- *Discounted Uusual, Customary, and Reasonable Rate (UCR):* A method that establishes for each service a provider reimbursement amount below the usual, customary, and reasonable charge for that service. Providers agree to accept discounted UCR in exchange for a guaranteed high volume of patients.

There are different types of managed care organizations, and hybrids continue to evolve as the market changes. Figure 6 is a brief description of the basic models. The distinctions between these different types often blur, however.

There is no definitive research on how managed care affects patient care [*National Journal* 1994]. Overall, there is little evidence to suggest that managed care either increases or decreases the number of physician visits, the use of preventive health care services, or in-patient hospital care [Rowland et al. 1995]. Yet there is no doubt that the switch to managed care will continue and will affect access to health care services and quality of care.

Managed care offers the potential for real improvements in patient care. In theory, it stresses prevention and can provide centralized services and more convenient hours. The financial incentives characteristic of MCOs may operate to reduce unnecessary or inappropriate prescription of services. On the other hand, they also have the potential to reduce the quality of medical care by denying patients beneficial treatments.

There is reason for concern that the construct of managed care may hinder health care treatment. Medical decisions are no longer made by doctors and patients alone. Now there is a third—and often

## Figure 6. Types of Managed Care Organizations

- Health maintenance organizations (HMOs) are capitated, prepaid health plans in which a selected group of providers offer preventive services and medical care. Each patient's care is managed by one case manager or gatekeeper. Staff model HMOs are usually nonprofit; they have their own clinical and lab facilities and full-time salaried staffs. Network HMOs include providers who contract with the HMO to provide certain services. HMOs often require enrollees to receive all of their care within the plan's network.

- Point-of-service plans (POSs) provide the bulk of services within a prepaid HMO but allow enrollees to use services outside the HMO in exchange for higher premiums and out-of-pocket payments.

- Preferred provider organizations (PPOs) allow enrollees to choose from a list of doctors and hospitals in their community. The PPO may review individual providers' treatment and care decisions and reimburse them according to rates negotiated by the service rather than through capitated payments. PPO members may choose out-of-plan providers but will be charged more for doing so.

- Independent practice associations (IPAs) are HMOs that contract with independent doctors and hospitals to provide care for their enrollees according to the treatment protocols, per-case fees, and review and approval rules set by the plan. Care is prepaid, and enrollees are covered only when they use HMO-designated providers and hospitals.

**Source:** Finkelstein, R. Hurwit, C., & Kirsch, R. (1995). The *managed care consumer's bill of rights.* New York: The Public Policy and Education Fund of New York, in Cooperation with the Citizens Fund.

pivotal—party to the decision making: the payor. Most HMOs use financial incentives in their compensation arrangements with physicians to encourage them to control the number of services they prescribe for plan enrollees (GAO 1995). The physician, often called a gatekeeper, coordinates care and limits unnecessary specialist visits, hospital stays, or lab tests.

While under traditional fee-for-service arrangements the financial incentive can result in too many services, MCOs offer providers financial incentives to provide too few. Some plans have utilization review or claims review personnel who police spending. Other plans reward doctors or hospitals for being conservative in their use of resources. Some require providers to stay within fixed budgets; others offer bonuses to doctors who keep spending within limits.

MCOs also may contain costs by limiting the choices among or denying access to providers with expertise in a particular disease or condition. An MCO could prohibit the use of specialists as primary care physicians or place arbitrary limits on some benefits, such as rehabilitation, home health, and mental health services. Some MCOs include confidentiality clauses that can discourage doctors from talking openly to patients about the need for specialty care and the role of managed care companies in limiting tests and treatments.

## Medicaid Managed Care

Medicaid is an extremely costly program for both federal and state governments. In the late 1980s and early 1990s, Medicaid expenditures increased dramatically as a result of extraordinary growth in health care costs, an expanding poverty population, and the rising cost of nursing home care for the low-income elderly. Although the rate of growth in Medicaid spending now has begun to drop, it continues to be a major budget consideration, prompting many states to seek waivers from federal regulations in order to experiment with nontraditional ways of providing health care to the poor. Increasingly, states are turning to managed care to provide access to high quality health care at a controllable cost. According to a 1996 HHS fact sheet, 32% of the total Medicaid population (almost 11.6 million people) were covered by managed care at the beginning of

1996. Enrollment in Medicaid managed care plans has increased 140% since January 1993. Currently, 49 states offer some form of managed care.

Under current law, a state that wishes to establish a Medicaid managed care program usually must obtain one of two types of waivers from the Health Care Financing Administration (HCFA) at HHS:

- *The Medicaid 1915(b) waiver* allows states to restrict beneficiaries' choice of provider by requiring enrollment in certain health plans, including managed care, or with certain providers.

- *The 1115 research and demonstration waiver* allows states to test broad changes, including revamping their entire Medicaid programs. States are using 1115 waivers to restructure eligibility, revise benefits, and mandate managed care for Medicaid beneficiaries.

There is growing pressure to allow states to move Medicaid recipients into managed care without going through any federal waiver process. Whether this happens or not, some of the greatest growth in managed care over the next few years likely will occur within the Medicaid program.

Some studies suggest that managed care can work reasonably well for the poor and improve access to primary care [Access 1995]. Before managed care, Medicaid was an insurance card and a promise to pay for services received. It did not guarantee the provision of services. Medicaid under managed care becomes a contractual obligation on the part of a provider to offer a set of health care services. This could mean that Medicaid recipients can access services more easily and truly benefit from this transformation of health care. There is evidence of numerous problems, however, in the ability of managed care to address the unusually serious and extensive health care needs of the Medicaid population.

Right now, MCOs are eager to contract with state Medicaid programs to provide care to Medicaid beneficiaries. The private health care arena is thought to be near saturation, while Medicaid is viewed as an untapped market. A real danger, however, is that an

MCO may not understand the complexities of serving this particular population. Medicaid recipients are a population in poorer health than privately ensured enrollees. They often are not seen by health care professionals until their conditions are so advanced as to require intensive, costly services. According to one study, serving AFDC Medicaid patients cost managed care plans nearly 25% more than serving their non-poor counterparts. Much of the excess cost is the result of hospitalization for illnesses that could have been managed in a lower-cost ambulatory care setting if diagnosed earlier [*Health Policy and Child Health* 1995].

Managed care is based on the premise that preventive and primary care for enrollees are good financial investments because they can prevent illnesses and lower health expenditures. Because Medicaid recipients often are enrolled for only short periods of time in any one health plan, MCOs may be unable to manage the health care needs of these patients properly and furnish the primary care they need to prevent serious illness. Plans therefore may have little incentive to pay enough for primary and preventive care or to invest in the expansion of primary care activities. Indeed, the incentives may be on underpaying for care—which in the case of Medicaid is already being furnished at a discounted rate—in order to realize a return—a problem significant in Medicaid fee-for-service care as well.

Although the needs of Medicaid patients often are greater than those of the general population, the ability of Medicaid patients to access the health care system is typically less. Medicaid recipients must receive information on all aspects of the managed care contract, including what services they are eligible for and how to change providers or appeal service decisions. In capitated systems, MCOs will get paid for the patients they enroll even if they never provide them care. For this reason, it is essential that outreach requirements be incorporated in all MCO contracts, especially for populations who are not sophisticated at maneuvering through the health care system or for whom health care is not a priority.

## Implications for Children in Foster Care

Although children make up 51% of all Medicaid users, they account for only 16% of all Medicaid expenditures. This is because most children are healthy and require very few specialty services—an ideal population for Medicaid. The exceptions to this are children in foster care and other children with special health care needs. Until now, states often have "carved out"—that is, exempted from mandatory managed care enrollment—these hard-to-serve, medically complicated populations. But children in foster care need to have their health managed. The existing fee-for-service system is cumbersome and confusing—especially for social workers and foster parents, who already struggle with too many demands and too little information.

As managed care becomes the prevalent system of health care, and more and more health resources are dedicated to managed care plans, these children need to be included. By the end of 1994, over three-fourths of all doctors were participating in managed care [Eckholm 1994]. In some places, it already is impossible to find providers who are not in MCO networks.

For children in foster care, the existing fee-for-service system of care has many problems. Conceivably, many of these problems could be well addressed by a managed care system. Managed care could ensure immediate access to health care services, complete health care screenings, and improved recordkeeping, and improve access to immunizations and preventive and primary care. The quality of care within MCOs can be assessed relatively easily, and accountability for care can be established and monitored. Ideally, MCOs could provide case management and an integrated, centralized, and coordinated system for children in foster care, who typically require multiple evaluation and treatment services from a variety of community providers [Simms & Halfon 1994]. Managed care could contain costs and use dollars spent on children in foster care more effectively than at present.

But for this to happen, there must be changes within the child welfare system. Managed care will be hard pressed to serve children in foster care well unless the child welfare system has the capacity to enroll these children, track them, and monitor their follow-up throughout their placement changes. Child welfare systems must obtain medical records and histories and forward them promptly to the MCO providers. Most importantly, child welfare workers must be advocates for children in foster care to be sure these children receive all the services they need. And equally important, departments of child welfare must be partners with the departments that administer Medicaid in detailing services, criteria, and protocols before contracts are negotiated with the MCOs. Credentialing must include adequate numbers of providers with the skills, knowledge, and background to manage the care of children and families in the foster care system.

Children with disabilities and chronic medical conditions do place great demands on health care systems. They require many more doctor visits and specialized services—including occupational therapy, physical therapy, and speech and language therapy—than typical children. In a capitated managed care environment, primary health care providers, at financial risk because of the children in their care, may have little incentive—and may, in fact, have disincentives—to refer a child for specialized care or supplemental services. Examinations of children in foster care are more time consuming than those for typical children because of their extensive health care needs and the psychological and social trauma they have experienced. In addition, physician time is required to coordinate cases with other providers, foster parents, and county and community agencies.

All children require the well-baby visits, immunizations, and other preventive and primary care services that managed care organizations typically provide so well. Children with special health needs and those in foster care can require much more extensive services. For this reason, managed care contracts must contain a broad and well-defined standard of medical necessity. MCOs are agents of state departments of health or medical assistance. It is the responsibility of these Medicaid offices to structure managed care contracts that meet the range and intensity of the health care needs of children in foster care, and to reimburse the MCOs accordingly.

"Not all managed care plans . . . have the capacity to offer the broad range of services available under Medicaid, and many do not have within their network the full range of providers that children need." [Newacheck et al. 1994].

# Conclusion

The trend for managed care is growth, especially in the public sector. States will continue to encourage, if not require, the shifting of Medicaid beneficiaries from traditional health care into lower-cost managed care plans. For this reason, it is critical for departments of child welfare to understand the revolution that is taking place in the delivery and financing of health care and its implications for the children they serve. Similarly state Medicaid agencies must consider the unique health, developmental, and social issues of children in foster care when negotiating managed care contracts on their behalf.

Managed care has the potential to effectively address the health care needs of children in foster care. If not appropriately designed and implemented, however, managed care can deprive these children of the services they so critically need. Managed care plans have limited experience in providing services for low-income children and serving children with complex medical and psychosocial problems. Many are designed for "normal risk" people and use restrictive medical necessity criteria. The financial incentives in managed care to limit services may collide with the complexities of serving a population like children in foster care. Likewise, careful attention must be paid to reimbursement rates so they take into account the special health service needs of children in foster care.

Because of the severity of their health problems and the inability of the existing fee-for-service system to serve them well, children in foster care may truly benefit from managed care. States may find that managed care can increase these children's access to and utilization of appropriate services while containing costs. But to make it work, departments of child welfare and Medicaid must partner to carefully consider all the variables and put together sensible approaches.

# References

Access for low-income, inner-city, minority populations: How has managed care affected the urban minority poor and essential community providers? (1995, August). *Health Policy and Child Health*. Adapted from a report originally prepared for The Commonwealth Fund by J. Darnell, S. Rosenbaum, L. Scarpulla-Nolan, A. Zuvekas, & P. Budetti. Washington, DC: George Washington University Center for Health Policy Research.

Eckholm, E. (1994, December 18). While Congress remains silent, health care transforms itself. *New York Times*, pp. A1, 34.

Finkelstein, R., Hurwit, C, & Kirsch, R. (1995, October). *The managed care consumer's bill of rights*. New York: The Public Policy and Education Fund of New York in cooperation with the Citizens Fund.

Newacheck, P., Hughes, D., Stoddard, J., & Halfon, N. (1994). Children with chronic illness and Medicaid managed care. *Pediatrics 93*, 497–500.

Rowland, D., Rosenbaum, S., Simon, L., & Chait, E. (1995, March). *Medicaid and managed care: Lessons from the literature*. Washington, DC: Kaiser Commission on the Future of Medicaid.

Simms, M.D., & Halfon, N. (1994, September–October). The health care needs of children in foster care: A research agenda. *Child Welfare LXXIII* (5), 505–524.

Unmanaged care? (1994, December 10). *National Journal 26* (50), 2903–2907.

U.S. Department of Health and Human Services (HHS). (1996, February). Fact sheet: Managed care in medicare and medicaid. Washington, DC: Author.

U.S. General Accounting Office (GAO). (1995, April). *Medicaid managed care: More competition and oversight would improve California's expansion plan*. Washington, DC: Author.

# Chapter Three

# Important Issues and Strategies for Care

With managed care still evolving and Medicaid forever on the federal and state chopping block, it is impossible to suggest all-encompassing, lasting solutions to the health care needs of children in foster care. Nonetheless, some specific recommendations can guide child welfare administrators and the managed care industry in designing managed care systems that will meet the needs of these children.

## Provider/Managed Care Organization Requirements

Given the substantial health problems of children in placement, the demands upon the primary health care provider are likely to be extensive. Children's health issues are different from those of adults and are most appropriately addressed by pediatricians. Pediatricians who care for children in the child welfare system must be trained for and comfortable with conducting physical-abuse examinations; collecting forensic evidence and testifying in civil and criminal court proceedings; conducting extensive and time-intensive health evaluations that include physical, emotional, and educational issues and an understanding of the child's legal and placement status; and communicating with the many people who share responsibility for the child, including social workers, the court, foster parents, and biological parents [Schor 1988].

## *Recommendations*

- Providers should be specialists in child health care and understand the special needs and circumstances of children in foster care.

- MCOs should have an adequate number of pediatric primary care providers with the proper qualifications and credentials to meet the needs of children in foster care.

- MCOs should provide evaluation criteria to be used in selecting providers.

- Child welfare agencies should identify physicians and other health care providers who have experience in treating children in foster care. Together, they should train other providers to treat these children.

## Reimbursement Mechanisms

A major factor affecting the likelihood that children in foster care will receive the full extent of services they require is the adequacy of reimbursement. When capitation is the reimbursement mechanism, the level at which capitation rates are set is critical.

The key tasks in setting an appropriate reimbursement rate are assessing the nature of the risk pool and weighing the rates for higher risk pools. For example, according to the National Association of Children's Hospitals and Related Institutions, 1% of the nation's children account for 37% of all health care costs for children. If MCOs were to capitate that 1%, the average annual cost would be $26,000; for the next 4% it would be $8,600; and for the next 95% it would be $315. Because the driving goal of states and MCOs is to reduce outlays for hospitals and other high-cost services, the greatest savings are likely to be with these high-cost patients. If payments offered by states or bid by MCOs are too low to cover necessary services, however, the quality of care may be jeopardized or the organization may collapse financially.

Typically, capitation rates are based on historical Medicaid data, which often underestimate true costs because of the traditional underservicing of children and the inappropriately low payments. To be accurate, this historical data must be supplemented with actual cost information.

MCOs will require higher reimbursement rates for children in foster care than for other children (possibly enhanced capitation, given the financial arrangement) in order to furnish the full range of services they require. Many children enter foster care with multiple unidentified health problems that will lead to high utilization at first, and possibly throughout the course of services.

## Recommendations

- States must set capitated rates at an amount that takes into account the increased costs associated with children in foster care given the composition of the risk pool. If the pool comprises the entire Medicaid population, including children in foster care, the capitation rate must be higher than if children in foster care are not included, but lower than if the pool comprised only children in foster care.

- The higher capitation fee must be passed on from the MCO to the provider.

- There must be a limit on the proportion of capitated fees that can be spent on administration and taken as profit.

- There must be a written protocol for the provision of services not covered in the MCO contract.

- There must be no copayments or other cost-sharing requirements for children in foster care.

- The state must retain responsibility for providing all the health care services children in foster care need that will not be covered in the MCO contract.

- There must be quality assurance and quality improvement mechanisms specific to children in foster care, with specified outcomes and monitoring processes. State agencies can use the information these mechanisms generate to guide recontracting decisions.

- The financial incentives for primary care gatekeepers to deny care must be minimized.

## Portability

Children in foster care move—from location to location, from one type of placement to another, sometimes from state to state, and in and out of their own homes. These moves can happen at any time of the month. Children may lose and regain Medicaid eligibility. If they are in an MCO with a limited geographic reach, they may move out of the coverage area.

### Recommendations

- There must be no lapses in coverage or waiting periods to receive medical care. Children in foster care cannot be restricted to usual designated enrollment periods.

- The child welfare agency must establish a health benefits coordinator, or ombudsperson, to ensure continuous health care coverage for children in foster care and to act as a liaison among plans and MCOs.

- The child welfare agency must be aware of the geographical areas covered by the MCO. If a child is placed outside the boundaries of the MCO, the agency must access Medicaid-reimbursed health care for the child through coordination with another MCO or through a fee-for-service system.

In some instances, an MCO can be responsible for access to health care providers outside its regular coverage area. It can use its commercial network or make arrangements to pay providers a fee for service until the child is enrolled in another HMO or returns to Medicaid fee-for-service care.

# Access to Services

Children in foster care need health care services when they enter care and throughout their stay in care. For many foster families, the lack of transportation to doctors and medical facilities can prove a real barrier to medical care. MCOs must be sensitive to the cultural diversity of children in foster care and foster families.

## *Recommendations*

- Services must be community based and accessible by public transportation, with convenient hours of operation.

- The maximum distance to both primary and specialty providers should generally be no more than 30 miles or 30 minutes. (This may not be possible with some types of specialty care for children who have special needs or disabilities.)

- Services must be culturally competent, with appropriate language competencies and an understanding of culturally-based health care practices.

- The child welfare agency must establish a health benefits coordinator, or ombudsperson, to advocate for patients and educate beneficiaries about new patterns of seeking service under managed care. Consumers need someone to help them thread their way through the bureaucracies of managed care.

- The child welfare agency must establish a system for the expeditious transfer of health records between managed care plans.

- The child welfare staff and foster parents must receive training in what managed care is and how to maneuver the system.

- The MCO must offer an educational brochure and a toll-free hotline—available seven days a week, 24 hours a day, 365 days a year—to help foster families enroll in and access managed care services, including information on the location and availability of network physicians and dentists.

## Confidentiality

MCOs should make providers aware of codes and statutes specific to children in foster care that relate to confidentiality.

### *Recommendations*

- Providers should be trained to understand the legal requirements regarding confidentiality and disclosure specific to children in foster care, develop procedures and documentation that clients can understand around release of information, and understand the legal and ethical consequences of violating a client's confidentiality.

- Providers should be trained to identify and report instances of child abuse and neglect.

- Agencies should work with MCOs to maximize sharing of information necessary to both professions.

## Benefit Packages

Children in foster care have a large number of unidentified medical problems and a wide range of often complex health care needs. Many have suffered severe physical and sexual abuse and have conditions that require complex diagnoses—including shaken baby syndrome, failure to thrive, subdural hematomas, and sexually transmitted diseases. Correct diagnosis is important not only so these children receive the treatment they need but also so they can be protected from further abuse. These children require a health care system that can address the totality of their needs. The EPSDT standard is broad, and appropriately reflects this range of needs. It ensures that children with congenital conditions, developmental delays, physical illnesses, and mental disabilities will receive the services they need to promote optimal development [Access 1995].

## *Recommendations*

- The services the MCO offers must be comprehensive; allow continuity with a primary care provider; and coordinate and integrate health, mental health, and developmental functions.

- The services provided to children in foster care must be sufficient in amount, duration, and scope to address their needs.

- The federally defined EPSDT range of services, modified to reflect current practices recommended by the American Academy of Pediatricians, must be included in all MCO contracts with the state.

- Each MCO serving children in foster care must have the capacity to perform forensic pediatric sexual abuse exams.

## Specialized Medical Services

Most children in out-of-home care need specialized care and assessments that go beyond the basics. They need specialist and subspecialist services, including access to pediatric HIV centers; PKU clinics; and programs for sickle cell anemia, drug and lead exposure, and other conditions. Children in foster care often have serious and extensive dental problems. Because so many children's disorders are relatively rare, many plans do not have pediatric specialists in their networks. A study by the American Academy of Pediatricians found that plans may discourage referrals to specialists or encourage patients to use in-plan providers who may have no training in the disorders that affect these children or their patterns of development [Cartland & Yudkowsky 1992].

## *Recommendations*

- The state must consider whether certain special-needs populations or certain specialized services should be "carved out" of the managed care contract.

- The state must consider whether certain special-needs populations should be "carved in" and provided specially tailored packages of services.

- MCOs must provide or arrange for specialized services in a con-
tinued and timely fashion. One strategy would be for the state
to require linkages with existing specialty and subspecialty care
providers or centers.

- Children in foster care must receive all services necessary to correct or ameliorate any medical or mental health conditions that
limit their daily functioning and well-being, without arbitrary
limitations.

- Services must include full dental coverage.

## Behavioral Health Services

The most frequently identified health problems of children in foster
care are emotional disorders. Children enter foster care because of
difficult conditions in the home environment, the profound consequences of which require continuing mental health attention
[CWLA 1988].

### Recommendations

- The state must consider whether behavioral health services
should be "carved out" of the managed care contracts.

- A wide range of behavioral health services must be available,
including routine screening and outpatient services, inpatient
services, and intermediate services such as day treatment. This
range should include individual, group, and family therapies.

- A variety of service delivery sites must be available, including
group homes and other community-based settings.

- Services must be available in the frequency and duration necessary
to address the behavioral health needs of children in foster care.

## Immediate Eligibility

Children entering the foster care system often need immediate health care as a result of abuse and neglect. Their conditions may be compounded by the emotional stress associated with removal from their families and placement in out-of-home care. Children entering foster care should receive pre-placement assessments—immediate physical exams. An initial screening can identify any health problems that require immediate treatment and alert foster parents and case-workers to other health conditions. Some states also require physicals when children move from one placement to another. The findings from these examinations help child welfare workers and the judicial system to plan appropriate interventions, treatments, and placements.

### Recommendations

- The department administering Medicaid must direct MCOs to allow instant eligibility for children in foster care, with no waiting periods before they receive medical services.

- There must be no preexisting condition exclusions.

- The child welfare system must appoint a health benefits coordinator, or ombudsperson, to enroll children in foster care in the MCO.

- The child welfare system must establish a system for the expeditious transfer of health records between managed care plans. MCOs are in a position to assist in this transfer-of-records process.

## Case Management

Case management involves coordinating all health care and ancillary services and often includes scheduling appointments and transportation to ensure that children receive the benefits of comprehensive health care. Case management can be provided in a number of ways. One effective approach is the development of a "medical home" for each child so the child has an ongoing relationship with a pediatric provider who coordinates his or her care [Simms & Halfon 1994]. Having a medical home reduces the trauma of establishing new health care relationships for a child who may be moving from placement to placement. The continuity of the health care provider can improve the overall quality of the assessment process by building a longitudinal perspective from which to evaluate changes in status. Some relatively subtle health or developmental problems may become known only after a prolonged period of observation.

*Recommendations*

- The child welfare agency, with the cooperation of the MCO, must implement a means to ensure the availability of key medical information and communication between health providers, biological parents, foster parents, and social workers.

- The MCO must assign each child in care to a pediatric provider, who will serve as the child's medical home.

- The child welfare or Medicaid agency must ensure that case management services are included in the benefits package. Otherwise, alternative methods for care coordination must be developed.

## Recordkeeping

The attempt to provide adequate medical care for children who enter the foster care system is often hampered by a lack of historical information and medical records.

*Recommendations*

- The child welfare system and the MCO each must keep centralized and coordinated records of current medical and psychosocial data in order to keep track of needs, services, gaps, and follow-through.

- The child welfare system and the MCO must agree on how and where information will be recorded and how it will be communicated to the people who need it, including the child's case worker, foster parents, and health care team.

- Redundancy in recordkeeping must be minimized.

## Quality Assurance and Quality Improvement

There is a need for mechanisms that make services predictable and accountable. There must be established standards of care, quality assurance monitoring, and assigned responsibility for oversight of care. The National Committee for Quality Assurance has developed a Medicaid Health Plan Employer Data and Information Set (HEDIS 3.0), performance measures specifically designed so health plans that serve Medicaid beneficiaries can measure managed care performance in meeting the special needs that may be present for the Medicaid population. HEDIS offers governments a first step in monitoring Medicaid managed care plans, providing feedback to the plans themselves, and eventually informing beneficiaries about the performance of competing plans. A later revision will reflect the specific needs of children in foster care.

### Recommendations

- The state should withhold a portion of the managed care fee until the MCO has complied with key contractual terms—for example, providing annual preventive care. This will give Medicaid an enforcement tool widely used in the private sector.

- The MCO must institute a readily accessible appeals process to address disagreements with the managed care company's decisions to deny services or referrals.

- The state should use HEDIS as a first-step performance measure for contract compliance and in making recontracting decisions. A stronger, more specific measure must be developed to evaluate the care of children in foster care.

## Prior Approval

Under many managed care systems, doctors have limited authority to make decisions about continuing care or make referrals for specialized care. For many services, they must get prior approval from the plan.

### *Recommendations*

- Prior-approval requirements should relate only to highly specialized or expensive services.

- Prior-approval requirements should be used only when there are requests for significant extensions of services.

- Prior-approval requirements must be waived when child welfare agencies are conducting child abuse and neglect investigations and require physical and sexual abuse examinations.

- MCOs should be required to approve or deny services within a specified and short period of time.

## Medical Necessity

Medical necessity is a standard that insurers or health plans, and Medicaid itself, use as the test of whether a covered service is actually needed by a patient under given circumstances. Whereas a benefits package lists what types of services are covered, the medical-necessity standard provides health plans and Medicaid with a benchmark for deciding—for a particular patient—the actual scope of services to be provided, in terms of both the level or intensity and the length of service.

Currently, the medical-necessity standard applies to all Medicaid services. The term is not defined in federal law and has become the subject of debate. Concerns often arise that medical necessity has been or will be too narrowly defined and that essential services will be denied.

## Recommendation

- The medical necessity standard of care must be defined to reflect the range of physical, psychosocial, and developmental problems that children in foster care experience.

# Social Necessity

Cases arise in which it may no longer be medically necessary for a child to be in a hospital but there are nonmedical reasons that she or he cannot be discharged. These include cases of abandoned children, boarder babies, or children on hospital protective service holds.

## Recommendation

- MCOs should be responsible for medical necessity days only. Arrangements must be made so that children are placed in appropriate settings quickly.

# State Pressure to Reduce Medicaid Costs

State budgets are squeezed by diminished federal contributions, demands for tax cuts, and the need to sustain infrastructure, schools, and care of the needy. States must be savvy consumers in negotiating with MCOs.

## Recommendations

- States must maximize their leverage as large purchasers of care to obtain good prices from health plans and providers. By asking providers and plans to bid on Medicaid and public employee health contracts jointly, states can lower prices while enrolling children in foster care in the same health plans that serve middle-class consumers.

- States should use market-based reforms—such as expanded risk pools—to purchase services efficiently, rather than denying essential health care to children and families.

## Contract Language

Medicaid managed care is based on a series of key contractual arrangements. The master contract is between the state (the Medicaid office) and the MCO. Subcontracts move the duties, responsibilities, and sometimes the risks down from the MCO to the provider networks. The MCO or the provider network may then subcontract with individual providers and facilities. These subcontracts move the duties; the responsibilities; and, again—if there is sub-capitation—the risks further down to the individual provider and facility.

There must be checks throughout the line of contracts to ensure that all services and expected outcomes are clearly described.

### Recommendations

- The requirements included in the master contract must be reflected in each level of subcontract.

- The contract language must guarantee that services provided to children in foster care are sufficient in amount, duration, and scope to address their needs.

- The plan must disclose the services for which each party is responsible at each level of contracting.

- Because some services will not be the responsibility of the plan, the state must explain in writing how it will provide these services. Such services could include long-term care, behavioral health care, and some kinds of medical equipment.

## Conclusion

Children in foster care have complex problems and require a broad range of physical health, mental health, and supplemental services to overcome the effects of abuse and neglect. Fitting these intense needs and complicated social circumstances into a changing American health care system is an awesome but doable task. This guide is meant to offer the information and direction that agencies need to ensure continuous, comprehensive health coverage for children in foster care.

# References

Access for low-income, inner-city, minority populations: How has managed care affected the urban minority poor and essential community providers? (1995, August). *Health Policy and Child Health.* Adapted from a report originally prepared for The Commonwealth Fund by J. Darnell, S. Rosenbaum, L. Scarpulla-Nolan, A. Zuvekas, & P. Budetti. Washington, DC: George Washington University Center for Health Policy Research.

Cartland, J.D.C., & Yudkowsky, B.K. (1992). Barriers to pediatric referral in managed care systems. *Pediatrics 89,* 183–192.

Child Welfare League of America (CWLA). (1988). *CWLA standards for health care services for children in out-of-home care.* Washington DC: Author.

Schor, E.L. (1988, December). Foster care. *The Pediatric Clinics of North America 35* (6), 1241–1252.

Simms, M.D., & Halfon, N. (1994, September–October). The health care needs of children in foster care: A research agenda. *Child Welfare LXXIII* (5), 505–524.

# *Appendix A*

# Medicaid Managed Care: The Experience So Far

## Positive results

- Emergency room visits decline.

- A mainstreaming effect occurs, with Medicaid-enrolled children's usual source of care often shifting to physicians' offices and away from clinics and hospital outpatient departments.

- A greater proportion of children rely on one provider, and substantially fewer use multiple providers.

- Use of routine preventive services—child health supervision services and immunizations—stays the same or slightly increases, according to early studies, although compliance stays below the recommended standards of the American Academy of Pediatrics [Fox et al. 1993].

- Inpatient hospital use is slightly lower.

- State Medicaid agencies usually mandate EPSDT preventive services and periodicity requirements.

## Problems encountered

- Contracts are not explicitly incorporating EPSDT benefits.

- State Medicaid agencies fail to insist on the EPSDT requirement for appropriate diagnostic and treatment services and medical necessity criteria.

- Contracts are using too narrow a medical necessity standard to determine whether a service is covered.

- States fail to clearly define "medically necessary Medicaid-covered services," so the plans define it for themselves.

- Subcontracts between MCOs and providers do not reflect the master contract between the state and the MCO.

- Managed care plans may restrict children's access to pediatricians and pediatric specialists.

- States do not set capitation rates high enough to take into account the increased service needs and costs of special-needs children.

- Managed care plans require prior authorization for specialty care services and then create financial disincentives for appropriate specialty care referrals.

- Managed care plans create financial incentives for physicians to limit patient visits in time and number.

- Difficulties in accessing services may increase. Barriers to care include transportation needs and language and cultural differences.

- Quality assurance mechanisms are inadequate.

- Cost savings are less than anticipated because of high administrative costs and high capitation rates in managed care programs.

- Lack of forceful state monitoring of Medicaid managed care organizations can lead to significant access and quality of care problems, including

- contracting with poor-quality providers,

- denial of needed emergency care,

- failure to provide appropriate specialty referrals,

- failure to provide required children's health screenings and treatment,

- failure to implement data collection and quality assurance systems,

- diversion of excessive dollars to administrative costs and profits.

- Plans may offer Medicaid enrollees a more limited network of providers than they offer commercial enrollees and place more stringent utilization controls on them.

- Some studies have found that poor children receive less preventive care in managed care plans than in fee-for-service plans [Families USA 1996].

- State HMO Medicaid payments are significantly lower that those made through the commercial market.

# References

Families USA. (1996). *Medicaid emergency tool kit: Managed care.* Washington, DC: Author.

Fox, H., McManus, M., & Leibowitz, A. (1993, February). *What we know about managed care for children.* Washington, DC: Child Health Consortium.

# *Appendix B*

# Checklist of Needed Services for Children in Foster Care

- Immediate eligibility for services.

- Seven-day-a-week, 24-hour-a-day emergency services.

- Community-based services.

- Culturally competent services, including language capacity that matches consumers' primary language.

- Initial health screening within 24 hours appropriate to the child's circumstances and agency concerns at the time the child enters foster care.

- Comprehensive, multidisciplinary health, mental health, and developmental assessment within one month of the child's placement [AAP 1994; CWLA 1989].

- Screening tests for common medical conditions, such as anemia or lead poisoning [Simms & Halfon 1994; AAP 1988], and risk assessments and screening tests for specialized conditions, including HIV and in utero drug exposure if indicated.

- Developmental and mental health evaluations on a regular schedule.

- Immunizations.

- Comprehensive dental services, including relief of pain and infection, restoration of teeth, and maintenance of dental health [CRS 1993].

- Follow-up diagnostic and treatment services for all conditions and problems identified in the health assessment and developmental and mental health evaluations.

- Covered costs of hearing aids, eyeglasses, and other equipment.

- Ongoing primary and preventive health care services, including reassessments at least every six months.

- Access to appropriate specialty and subspecialty care.

- Case management that designates one individual or center to be responsible for coordinating all aspects of the health care of each foster child, including a plan to meet the child's health care needs and identification of responsibilities and recommendations for follow-up care. Case management services must include assistance with scheduling appointments and transportation.

- Coordinated medical and psychosocial recordkeeping.

## Sources

American Academy of Pediatrics (AAP), Committee on Psychosocial Aspects of Child and Family Health. (1988). Guidelines for health supervision II. Elk Grove Village, IL: Author.

American Academy of Pediatrics (AAP) Committee on Early Childhood Adoption and Dependent Care. (1994, February). Health care of children in foster care. *Pediatrics 93* (2), 1–4.

Child Welfare League of America (CWLA). (1989). *Standards for service for abused or neglected children and their families.* Washington, DC: Author.

Congressional Research Service (CRS). (1993, January). *Medicaid source book: Background data and analysis. A report prepared for the Committee on Energy and Commerce, U.S. House of Representatives.* Washington, DC: Author.

Simms, M.D., & Halfon, N. (1994, September–October). The health care needs of children in foster care: A research agenda. *Child Welfare LXXIII* (5), 505–524.

# *Appendix C*

## Tasks for State Medicaid Offices

In negotiating MCO contracts, state Medicaid offices are mindful that all children have health needs different from those of adults. There are expected patterns of growth and development that must be monitored and assessed for needed interventions.

Children in foster care have the same health needs as children in the general population, as well as certain unique needs. Their lives are tumultuous, their physical and mental health often are poor, and their living conditions can be unstable. They often have complex problems and require a broad range of physical, mental health, and supplemental services to overcome the effects of abuse and neglect. They need health care providers who understand their particular situations and are willing and able to work with the courts, the agencies, and their caregivers. They need easy access to specialty care.

State Medicaid offices must consider children in foster care as a special and high-needs population. Managed care plans must be alerted to the gravity and extent of these children's health care problems and held accountable for their care. In return, MCOs and their providers must be compensated appropriately.

State Medicaid and child welfare offices must partner on behalf of children in foster care.

### Questions to Be Answered

- Is it possible to structure a Medicaid managed care program to meet the needs of children in foster care? If it is not possible to serve these children well through this system, can they be excluded from mandatory managed care and assured appropriate and comprehensive fee-for-service care?

- Will the MCO ensure access to medically necessary physical health, emotional health, and developmental services that children in foster care require?

- How will the MCO generate cost savings—from greater efficiencies or from denial of necessary care?

- Are there adequate numbers of primary care physicians within the MCO network who understand and can respond effectively to the needs of children in foster care?

- Will the MCO ensure that referrals are made to children's medical centers and other health care specialists?

- What quality-of-care standards for children are applied in the managed care program? How is *quality* defined, and by whom?

- What outcome measures will be used as indicators of effective care for children in foster care, particularly in the areas of mental health and developmental services?

- How will the state maintain effective oversight?

- Is the contract with the MCO specific, understandable, unambiguous, and enforceable? Does the contract articulate what constitutes breach and what the consequences and sanctions for breach will be? Is this also true of any and all devolving contracts?

- If a child must change MCOs, will continuous coverage be maintained? How will the medical records be transferred?

- What services are not included in the MCO contract, and how will these services be provided?

- Is there training for the MCO, physicians, and other health care providers on the unique needs and circumstances of children in foster care?

# Appendix D

## Tasks for Public Child Welfare Agencies

Child welfare agencies must follow the transformation of health care in their states. Agency administrators and staff members must understand the inevitable tendency of managed care to contain costs as aggressively as possible, which may lead to avoiding giving care or making it difficult for those in their care to get attention. They must alert the Medicaid office to the complex needs of children in foster care and to the state's responsibility for their care. Appropriate health care for children in the child welfare system can mean less time in foster care—a moral and financial incentive.

Child welfare agencies must be at the table as states consider any change in Medicaid, particularly when children in out-of-home care may be included within managed care. Their overriding question must be: How will this impact the health and well-being of these children? Child welfare professionals must ensure that managed care arrangements are designed to meet the unique health and service delivery needs of children in foster care. They should expect MCO contracts to include the full range of benefits these children need, and then they must see that the plans are held accountable for the services they are being paid to deliver.

For their part, child welfare agencies must have clear and streamlined processes in place to authorize routine health care so that services are not delayed. These processes may include empaneling a medical review board to assist with decisions involving experimental treatment, subjecting children to research protocols, termination of life support or do-not-resuscitate orders, and consent for treatment when biological parents refuse. Agencies must train foster parents and caseworkers to understand and utilize managed care, and provide an ombudsperson to help them with enrollment and advocacy on behalf of the children.

Child welfare agencies must be sure that all the services that children in foster care need are either covered in the managed care contract or the acknowledged responsibility of a state agency. This will mean sharing the financial responsibilities for the full range of services children need.

## Questions to Be Answered

- Is confidentiality appropriately safeguarded?

- Is confidentiality a barrier to serving children adequately?

- Do providers in the network have expertise in the area of child development and behavior? Child abuse and neglect?

- Is the MCO being reimbursed appropriately for this high-risk population?

- Will the state Medicaid office monitor the MCOs' reimbursement structures for providers?

- How will providers be paid: capitation, fee schedule, or other method?

- If payment is through capitation, are services fully or partially capitated?

- Does the contract ensure that services provided to children in foster care will be sufficient in amount, duration, and scope to address their needs?

- Does the plan maintain the full scope of diagnostic and treatment services federally allowable under EPSDT?

- Will the MCOs include all necessary services, such as substance abuse treatment, mental health services, ob-gyn care, primary medical care, transportation, case management, prevention counseling, home care, dental services, and long-term care?

• What services are not covered in the MCO contract?

• General questions to establish an understanding of the procedures:

  – What type of managed care waiver is the state seeking?

  – Within the waiver being sought, what departures from federal Medicaid law is the state proposing?

  – What population groups will be included within the waiver?

  – Does the waiver require approval by the state legislature? [Perkins & Rivera 1995]

• How is *emergency* defined in the contract? Are there retroactive denials of care?

• Who will pay for emergency services?

• Can out-of-plan emergency services be provided without prior approval?

• Is case management included and defined in the contract?

• What are the state Medicaid office's defined standards for *medical necessity* and *usual and customary* that will apply to all plans?

• On what basis can plans deny or limit services?

• Can participating providers subcontract with other providers for services?

• Are these subcontractors held to the same quality, accessibility, and reporting standards as contracting providers?

• How are geographical barriers handled?

- How is a child in foster care enrolled and disenrolled?

- Is there portability of coverage?

- Is there out-of-area coverage?

- What are the performance and outcome measures? Do they include components specific to the care of children in foster care—for example, percentage of a plan's children receiving required screens?

- What is the grievance procedure?

- What physicians and what facilities and providers are in the MCO network?

- Do the plans include providers specifically experienced in serving children in foster care?

- Are there copayments or other cost-sharing requirements?

- Are there maximum waiting times to obtain an appointment—same day, immediate, 30-day assessment, other?

- Do providers comply with requests for documentation to assist social service and legal actions on behalf of the children?

- Are services satisfactory to social workers, foster parents, and other health care providers?

# Reference

Perkins, J., & Rivera, L. (1995, July). *Medicaid managed care: 20 questions to ask your state.* San Francisco: National Health Law Program.

# For Further Reading

Access for low-income, inner-city, minority populations: How has managed care affected the urban minority poor and essential community providers? (1995, August). Health Policy and Child Health. Adapted from a report originally prepared for The Commonwealth Fund by J. Darnell, S. Rosenbaum, L. Scarpulla-Nolan, A. Zuvekas, & P. Budetti. Washington, DC: George Washington University Center for Health Policy Research.

American Academy of Pediatrics (AAP), Committee on Child Health Financing. (1995, April). Guiding principles for managed care arrangements for the health care of infants, children, adolescents, and young adults. *Pediatrics 95* (4), 613–615.

American Academy of Pediatrics (AAP), Committee on Child Health Financing. (1995). Purchasing quality pediatric care in commercial managed care plans (pamphlet).

American Academy of Pediatrics (AAP), Committee on Early Childhood Adoption and Dependent Care. (1994, February). Health care of children in foster care. *Pediatrics 93* (2), 1–4.

American Academy of Pediatrics (AAP), Committee on Psychosocial Aspects of Child and Family Health. (1988). *Guidelines for health supervision II.* Elk Grove Village, IL: Author.

American Public Welfare Association (APWA). (1990). *A commitment to change: Report of the National Commission on Child Welfare and Family Preservation.* Washington, DC: Author.

Barbell, K. (1995). *Foster care today: A briefing paper.* Washington, DC: Child Welfare League of America.

Barbell, K. (1996, March). Foster Care F.Y.I. #1. Washington, DC: Child Welfare League of America.

Bazelon Center for Mental Health. (1995, November). *Managing managed care for publicly financed mental health services.* Washington, DC: Author.

Blatt, S., Deitch, S., English, K., & Simms, M. (1996, January 23). *Health care for children in foster care.* Presentation at San Diego Child Maltreatment Conference.

Burden, L. (1994, May 2). Health care for children in foster care and the transition to Medi-Cal managed care. Sacramento: California Partnership for Children.

Cartland, J.D.C., & Yudkowsky, B.K. (1992). Barriers to pediatric referral in managed care systems. *Pediatrics 89,* 183–192.

Chernoff, R., Combs-Orme, T., Risley-Curtiss, C., & Heisler, A. (1994, April). Assessing the health status of children entering foster care. *Pediatrics 93* (4), 594–601.

Child Welfare League of America (CWLA). (1988). *CWLA standards for health care services for children in out-of-home care.* Washington DC: Author.

Child Welfare League of America (CWLA). (1989). *Standards for service for abused or neglected children and their families.* Washington DC: Author.

Child Welfare League of America (CWLA), North American Commission on Chemical Dependency and Child Welfare. (1992). *Children at the front: A different view of the war on alcohol and drugs.* Washington, DC: Author.

Children's Defense Fund. (1996, January 26). Medicaid for children and families: Actions to take in the states [On-line]. Available: HandsNet Forums/Health Issues/Medicaid.

Children's Research Institute of California. (1996). *The impact of managed care on foster children: An examination of the Sacramento geographic managed care system.* Sacramento: Author.

Citizens' Committee for Children, (1994). *Finding a way through the labyrinth: Medicaid managed care for children in southwest Brooklyn.* New York: Author.

Congressional Research Service (CRS). (1993, January). *Medicaid source book: Background data and analysis. A report prepared for the Committee on Energy and Commerce, U.S. House of Representatives.* Washington, DC: Author.

DeWoody, M. (1994). *Making sense of federal dollars: A funding guide for social service providers.* Washington, DC: Child Welfare League of America.

DeWoody, M., Barker, R., & Gnessin, A. *A primer on managed care: A guide for child welfare services providers.* Washington, DC: Child Welfare League of America. n.d.

DeWoody, M., Ceja, K., & Sylvester, M. (1993). *Independent living services for youths in out-of-home care.* Washington, DC: Child Welfare League of America.

Eckholm, E. (1994, December 18). While Congress remains silent, health care transforms itself. *New York Times,* A1, 34.

Emenhiser, D., Barker, R., & DeWoody, M. (1995). *Managed care: An agency guide to surviving and thriving.* Washington, DC: Child Welfare League of America.

Families USA. (1996). *Medicaid emergency tool kit: Managed care.* Washington, DC: Author.

Finkelstein, R., Hurwit, C., & Kirsch, R. (1995, October). *The managed care consumers' bill of rights.* New York: Public Policy and Education Fund of New York, in cooperation with the Citizens Fund.

Flaherty, E.G., & Weiss, H. (1990, March). Medical evaluation of abused and neglected children. *American Journal of Diseases of Children 144,* 330–334.

Fox, H., McManus, M., & Leibowitz, A. (1993, February). *What we know about managed care for children.* Washington, DC: Child Health Consortium.

Freudenheim, M. (1994, September 6). To economists, managed care is no cure-all. *New York Times,* pp. A1, A17.

Goerge, R.M., Wulczyn, F.H., & Harden, A.W. (1994). *Foster care dynamics 1983–1992: A report from the multistate foster care data archive.* Chicago: Chapin Hall Center for Children at the University of Chicago.

Halfon, N., Berkowitz, G., & Klee, L. (1992a. ). Children in foster care in California: An examination of medicaid reimbursed health services utilization. *Pediatrics 89*, 1230–1237.

Halfon, N., Berkowitz, G., & Klee, L. (1992b). Mental health service utilization by children in foster care in California. *Pediatrics 89*. 1238–1244.

Halfon, N., Berkowitz, G., & Klee, L. (1993). Development of an integrated case management program for vulnerable children. *Child Welfare LXXII* (4), 379–396.

Halfon, N., Mendonca, A., Berkowitz, G. (1995, April). Health status of children in foster care. *ARCH Pediatric Adolescent Medicine 149*, 386–392.

Hancock, E. (1995, November). The squeeze is on. *Johns Hopkins Magazine*, 48–55.

Hershowitz, J., Seck, M., & Fogg, C. (1989, June). *Substance abuse and family violence.* Boston: Massachusetts Department of Social Services.

Hochstadt, N., Jaudes, P., Zimo, D., & Schachter, J. (1987). The medical and psychosocial needs of children entering foster care. *Child Abuse and Neglect 11*, 3–62.

Hochstadt, N., & Yost, D. (Eds.). (1991). *The medically complex child: The transition to home care.* New York: Harwood Academic Publishers.

Horvath, J., & Kaye, N. (Eds.). (1995, May). *Medicaid managed care: A guide for states,* 2nd ed. Portland, ME: National Academy for State Health Policy.

Horwitz, S.M., Simms, M., & Farrington, R.M. (1994, April). Impact of developmental problems on young children's exits from foster care. *Journal of Developmental and Behavioral Pediatrics 15* (2), 105–110.

Kadushin, A., & Martin, J. A. (1988). *Child welfare services* (4th ed.). New York: Macmillan.

Kaiser Commission on the Future of Children. (1995, December). *Medicaid Facts.* Washington, DC: Author.

Kavaler, F., & Swire, M.R. (1972, November). Health services for foster children: An approach to evaluation. *Child Welfare LI* (9), 574-583.

Kavaler, F., & Swire, M. R. (1983). *Foster-child health care.* Lexington, MA: D.C. Heath and Co.

Klee, L., & Halfon, N. (1987). Mental health care for foster children in California. *Child Abuse and Neglect 11*, 63–74.

Larson, L. (1995, November). Pediatrician streamlines foster children's care. *AAP News*, 22–23.

Lindsay, S., Chadwick, D., Landsverk, J., & Pierce, E. (1993, November–December). A computerized health and education passport for children in out-of-home care: The San Diego model. *Child Welfare LXXII* (6), 581–593.

McManus, M., Fox, H., Newacheck, P., McPherson, M., & Roy, B. (1996, March). *Strengthening partnerships between state programs for children with special health needs and managed care organizations.* Washington, DC: Maternal and Child Health Policy Research Center.

Merkel-Holguin, L. (1993). *The child welfare stat book 1993.* Washington, DC: Child Welfare League of America.

Moffatt, M.E.K., Peddie, M., Stulginskas, J., et al. (1985). Health care delivery to foster children: A study. *Health and Social Work 10*, 129–137.

Molin, R. (1988). Treatment of children in foster care: Issues of collaboration. *Child Abuse and Neglect 12,* 241–249.

National Association of Children's Hospitals and Related Institutions. Choosing a health care plan for your child: A parent's guide. Alexandria, VA: Author. Pamphlet, n.d.

National Association of Children's Hospitals and Related Institutions. Understanding the basics of managed care: A parent's guide. Alexandria, VA: Author. Pamphlet, n.d.

National Commission on Children. (1991). *Beyond rhetoric: A new American agenda for children and families.* Washington, DC: Author.

National Foster Parent Association (NFPA). (1994, May). A survey of the states 1994. A report at the 1994 NFPA national conference.

Newacheck, P., Hughes, D., Stoddard, J., & Halfon, N. (1994). Children with chronic illness and Medicaid managed care. *Pediatrics 93,* 497–500.

Ooms, T. (1990). *The crisis in foster care: New directions for the 1990s.* Washington, DC: Family Impact Seminars. (Background briefing report and meeting highlights).

Open Minds. (1996). *Behavioral health risk-based and capitation contracting.* Gettysburg, PA: Author.

Oregon Department of Human Resources, Children's Services Division. (1995). *The Oregon health plan and you: A guide for foster parents.* Salem, OR: Author.

Oregon Department of Human Resources, Office of Medical Assistance Programs. (1996, March). *The Oregon Health Plan.* Salem, OR: Author.

Oregon Department of Human Resources, State Office for Services to Children and Families. (1996). *The OHP cookbook.* Salem, OR: Author.

Oss, M., & Mackie, J. J. (1995, December). Public managed behavioral health models. *Open Minds 9* (9).

Pearson, G. S. (1984, March). The development of mental health consultation to a foster care placement agency. *Public Health Nursing 1* (1).

Perkins, J., & Rivera, L. (1995, July). *Medicaid managed care: 20 questions to ask your state.* San Francisco: National Health Law Program.

Rosenbaum, S. (1996, January 20). *Managed care contracting under Medicaid.* Washington, DC: Center for Health Policy Research, George Washington University Medical Center.

Rowland, D., Rosenbaum, S., Simon, L., & Chait, E. (1995, March). Medicaid and managed care: Lessons from the literature. Washington, DC: Kaiser Commission on the Future of Medicaid.

Schor, E.L. (1979, November 5). An HMO for a high-risk population—foster children. Paper presented at the annual meeting of the American Public Health Association, New York, NY.

Schor, E.L. (1981, May). Health care supervision of foster children. *Child Welfare LV* (5), 313–319.

Schor, E.L. (1982, May). The foster care system and the health status of foster children. *Pediatrics 69* (5), 521–528.

Schor, E.L. (1988, December). Foster care. *The Pediatric Clinics of North America 35* (6), 1241–1252.

Schor, E.L. (1989, January). Foster care. *Pediatrics in Review* 10 (7), 209–216.

Schor, E.L., Neff, J. M., & LaAsmar, J. L. (1984, September–October). The Chesapeake Health Plan: An HMO model for foster children. *Child Welfare LXIII* ( 5), 431–440.

Simms, M.D. (1989). The foster care clinic: A community program to identify treatment needs of children in foster care. *Journal of Developmental and Behavioral Pediatrics 10*, 121–128.

Simms, M.D. (1991, August). Foster children and the foster care system, Part I: History and legal structure. *Pediatrics 21* (7), 297–321.

Simms, M.D. (1991, September). Foster children and the foster care system, Part II: Impact on the child. *Pediatrics 21* (8), 345–369.

Simms, M. D., & Halfon, N. (1994, September–October). The health care needs of children in foster care: A research agenda. *Child Welfare LXXIII* (5), 505–524.

Simms, M.D., & Kelly, R.W. (1991, July–August). Pediatricians and foster children. *Child Welfare LXX* (4), 451–461.

Takayama, J. (1994). Children in foster care in the state of Washington: Health care utilization and expenditures. *Journal of the American Medical Association 271* (23).

Tatara, T. (1993, October). *Characteristics of children in substitute and adoptive care*. Washington, DC: American Public Welfare Association, Voluntary Cooperative Information System.

Tatara, T. (1994, October). *Characteristics of children in substitute and adoptive care*. Washington, DC: American Public Welfare Association, Voluntary Cooperative Information System.

Taylor-Brown, S., Wilcyzinski, C., Moore, E., & Cohen, F. (1992). Perinatal AIDS: Permanency planning for the African American community. *Journal of Multicultural Social Work 2* (3), 85–100.

Unmanaged care? (1994, December 10). *National Journal 26* (50), 2903–2907.

U.S. Department of Health and Human Services (HHS). (1996, February). Fact sheet: Managed care in medicare and medicaid. Washington, DC: Author.

U.S. Department of Health and Human Services (HHS), Administration for Children and Families, Children's Bureau. (1993, August). *Report to Congress: National estimates on the number of boarder babies, the cost of their care, and the number of abandoned infants.* Washington, DC: Government Printing Office.

U.S. Department of Health and Human Services (HHS), National Center on Child Abuse and Neglect. (1995). *Child maltreatment 1993: Reports from the states to the National Center on Child Abuse and Neglect.* Washington, DC: Government Printing Office.

U.S. Department of Health and Human Services, National Center on Child Abuse and Neglect. (1996). *Child maltreatment 1994: Reports from the states to the National Center on Child Abuse and Neglect.* Washington, DC: Government Printing Office.

U.S. General Accounting Office (GAO). (1994, April). *Foster care: Parental drug abuse has alarming impact on young children.* Washington, DC: Author. (GAO/HEHS-94-89)

U.S. General Accounting Office (GAO). (1995, April). *Medicaid managed care: More competition and oversight would improve California's expansion plan.* Washington, DC: Author.

U.S. General Accounting Office (GAO). (1995, May). Foster care: Health needs of many young children are unknown and unmet. Washington, DC: Author (GAO/HEHS-95-114).

U.S. House of Representatives, Select Committee on Children, Youth, and Families. (1989, November). *No place to call home: Discarded children in America*. Washington, DC: U.S. Government Printing Office.

White, R., & Benedict, M. (1986, April). Health status and utilization patterns of children in foster care: Executive summary Authors.

White, R., Benedict, M., & Jaffe, S. (1987, September–October). Foster child health care supervision policy" *Child Welfare LXVI* (5), 387–398.

Youth Law Center, National Center for Youth Law. (1995). *Preventive health care for children: Medi-Cal managed care and EPSDT services*. San Francisco,: Author.

Yudkowsky, B.K., Cartland, J.D.C., & Flint, S.S. (1990). Pediatrician participation in Medicaid: 1978 to 1989. *Pediatrics 85,* 567–577.

# The CWLA National Advisory Committee on Managed Health Care for Children in Foster Care

BOB BARKER, M.S.W.
Executive Director
*Southwest Behavioral Healthcare Inc.*

STEVE BLATT, M.D.
Director
*ENHANCE Services for Children in Foster Care*
*State University of New York*
*Health Sciences Center*

FRED CHAFFEE
Executive Director
*Arizona Children's Home*

PATRICK CHAULK, M.D.
Senior Associate
*Annie E. Casey Foundation*

ABIGAIL ENGLISH, J.D.
Project Director
*National Health Care Project*
*National Center for Youth Law*

HARRIETTE B. FOX
President
*Fox Health Policy Consultants*

MADELYN DEWOODY FREUNDLICH, J.D.,
M.S.W., M.S.P.H.
Director
*The Adoption Institute Spence-Chapin Services*
*to Families and Children*

NEAL HALFON, M.D., M.P.H.
*School of Public Health and Medicine*
*University of California*

MS. LUCILLE MCCLUNEY
Foster Parent
*Branch Chief for Policy Review and Operations*
*U.S. Children's Bureau*

Beatrice Moore
*Deputy for Lashawn General Receivership*
*District of Columbia*

LAVDENA ORR, M.D.
*Director*
*Division of Child Protection*
*Children's National Medical Center*

MONICA OSS
President
*OPEN MINDS, Inc.*

EDWARD L. SCHOR, M.D.
Medical Director
*Division of Family and Community Health*
*Iowa Department of Public Health*

MARK SIMMS, M.D.
Director
*Child Development Center*
*Children's Hospital of Wisconsin*

JAKE TERPSTRA, M.S.W.
Licensing, Residential Care and
Child Welfare Specialist
*U.S. Children's Bureau*

CLEO TERRY, M.S.W.
Vice President
Child and Family Services
*Lifelink Corporation/*
*Bensenville Home Society*

KAY DEAN TORAN
Director,
*State Office for Services to Children and Families*
*Oregon Department of Human Resources*

ELIZABETH WEHR, J.D.
*Center for Health Policy Research*
*George Washington University*

WINIFRED WILSON
*Director, Maryland Commission for Families*

## CWLA Staff

KATHY BARBELL
Program Director
*Family Foster Care*

ELLEN BATTISTELLI
Senior Policy Analyst
*Project Director*

CHARLOTTE MCCULLOUGH
Director
Managed Care Institute

KARABELLE PIZZIGATI
Director of Public Policy

LYDIA RUSSO
Public Policy Assistant

BRUCE WEBB
Senior Consultant

Gratitude is an emotion that comes from appreciation. It's an awareness, a thankfulness of the good things in your life, in you and in the world around you. Gratitude is a powerful thing. It can turn any negative into a positive. It can change how you feel inside. It can bring hope and happiness. It can improve your health, your relationships, your career and so much more. It can literally transform your life.

So often in today's society, the negative is sensationalized and the positive is ignored. You see it in the news, in magazines and newspapers. You hear it in the grocery store, at work and even from family and friends. All of this negativity can be overwhelming to the point of wearing a person down.

If you're feeding into the negativity. If you're focusing on the negative rather than the positive, you are doing yourself a serious disservice. You are harming your emotional wellbeing as well as your physical body. You could be straining your relationships, hurting your career and much more.

When you express gratitude, it diminishes the negativity in a powerful way. Studies show that practicing gratitude leads to:

- A feeling of optimism, joy and satisfaction.
- Less stress, anxiety and depression.
- A strengthened immune system.
- Lower blood pressure.
- The ability to bounce back quicker after a traumatic event.
- Stronger relationships.
- A feeling of being connected to your community.
- Feeling less victimized by others or by life.
- Being able to recognize and appreciate what you have rather than what you don't.
- You becoming more compassionate and empathetic.
- A better quality and more rewarding life.

Practicing gratitude changes your perspective on life.

## Practicing Gratitude

In order to change your perspective, you need to make practicing gratitude a habit. One of the easiest, and most effective ways to do this is to keep a journal of the things you are grateful for.

Whether you choose to journal in the morning, or at night, or both is up to you. Pick a quiet time and spend a few minutes thinking about, documenting and appreciating the positive things in your life.

Writing in your journal every day will ensure you stay focused on the positive so the negative can be washed away. Do it for a month, two months, six months or more. The longer you do it, the more ingrained it will become in your mind and the more your thoughts will shift.

At first, recognizing the positive aspects may feel awkward, but the more you look for it, the more you will find. There is beauty all around you. There is beauty within you. A smile, a sunset, a friend, a personal goal being met. These are all things you can be grateful for. Even if you only find one thing to be grateful for each day, that's okay. It's a start. As you journal, try to work up to three, five or even ten things a day when possible.

The following pages can be printed as your first gratitude journal. It contains 10 prompts to get you started along with some quotes to keep you motivated. There is no right or wrong way to practice gratitude. The practice itself is where the power resides.

Think about a recent hardship. What positive aspect or opportunity came from it?

⌇

# List five things you love about yourself and why.

~⌒~

Write about a time when you really felt appreciative of something or someone in your life.

~

There's Always Something to Be Thankful For

# Write about your favorite season.

Think back to the past year or two. Write about some of the changes you've made and why you are grateful for them.

⁓

# Write about something you love doing and why you are grateful to be able to do it.

# List five positive aspects of your community and why you love them.

⌇

# Sunrise or Sunset? Which is your favorite and why?

# Write about how you felt the last time someone did a kind deed for you.

# Write about something that makes you belly laugh.

There's Always Something to Be Thankful For

"Saying thank you is more than good manners. It is good spirituality. "
~ Alfred Painter

‎

There's Always Something to Be Thankful For

There's Always Something to Be Thankful For

There's Always Something to Be Thankful For

There's Always Something to Be Thankful For

"Gratitude turns what we have into enough. "

___

There's Always Something to Be Thankful For

There's Always Something to Be Thankful For

There's Always Something to Be Thankful For

There's Always Something to Be Thankful For

There's Always Something to Be Thankful For

"God gave you a gift of 86,400 seconds today. Have you used one to say "thank you?" ~ William A. Ward

There's Always Something to Be Thankful For

There's Always Something to Be Thankful For

There's Always Something to Be Thankful For

*"Silent gratitude isn't much use to anyone." ~ Gertrude Stein*

_____

_____

_____

_____

_____

_____

_____

_____

_____

_____

_____

_____

_____

_____

_____

_____

_____

_____

_____

*There's Always Something to Be Thankful For*

There's Always Something to Be Thankful For

There's Always Something to Be Thankful For

There's Always Something to Be Thankful For

There's Always Something to Be Thankful For

"If the only prayer you said in your whole life was, "thank you," that would suffice." ~ Meister Eckhart

There's Always Something to Be Thankful For

There's Always Something to Be Thankful For

There's Always Something to Be Thankful For

There's Always Something to Be Thankful For

"If you count all your assets, you always show a profit." ~ Robert Quillen

There's Always Something to Be Thankful For

There's Always Something to Be Thankful For

There's Always Something to Be Thankful For

There's Always Something to Be Thankful For

"There are two kinds of gratitude – The sudden kind when we receive and the deeper kind when we give. "

~

There's Always Something to Be Thankful For

There's Always Something to Be Thankful For

There's Always Something to Be Thankful For

There's Always Something to Be Thankful For

"The struggle ends when the gratitude begins." ~ Neale Donald Walsch

There's Always Something to Be Thankful For

There's Always Something to Be Thankful For

There's Always Something to Be Thankful For

There's Always Something to Be Thankful For

There's Always Something to Be Thankful For

"Replace fear with gratitude, and the whole world changes."
~ Terri Guillemets

There's Always Something to Be Thankful For

There's Always Something to Be Thankful For

There's Always Something to Be Thankful For

There's Always Something to Be Thankful For

## "Hem your blessings with thankfulness so they don't unravel. "

There's Always Something to Be Thankful For

There's Always Something to Be Thankful For

There's Always Something to Be Thankful For

There's Always Something to Be Thankful For

"Gratitude is the memory of the heart." ~ Jean Baptiste Massieu

There's Always Something to Be Thankful For

There's Always Something to Be Thankful For

There's Always Something to Be Thankful For

There's Always Something to Be Thankful For

"Some people grumble that roses have thorns. I am grateful
that thorns have roses." ~ Alphonse Karr

There's Always Something to Be Thankful For

There's Always Something to Be Thankful For

There's Always Something to Be Thankful For

There's Always Something to Be Thankful For

"As we express our gratitude, we must never forget that the highest appreciation is not to utter words, but to live by them." ~ John F. Kennedy

_____

_____

_____

_____

_____

_____

_____

_____

_____

_____

_____

_____

_____

_____

_____

There's Always Something to Be Thankful For

There's Always Something to Be Thankful For

There's Always Something to Be Thankful For

There's Always Something to Be Thankful For

"We make a living by what we get, but we make a life by what we give."
~ Winston Churchill "

There's Always Something to Be Thankful For

There's Always Something to Be Thankful For

There's Always Something to Be Thankful For

There's Always Something to Be Thankful For

"It is impossible to feel grateful and depressed in the same moment."
~ Naomi Williams

There's Always Something to Be Thankful For

There's Always Something to Be Thankful For

There's Always Something to Be Thankful For

There's Always Something to Be Thankful For

There's Always Something to Be Thankful For

"Kindness is a language, which the deaf can hear and the blind can see."
~ Mark Twain

There's Always Something to Be Thankful For

There's Always Something to Be Thankful For

There's Always Something to Be Thankful For

There's Always Something to Be Thankful For

"Be thankful for what you have, you'll end up having more."
~ Oprah Winfrey

There's Always Something to Be Thankful For

There's Always Something to Be Thankful For

There's Always Something to Be Thankful For

There's Always Something to Be Thankful For

"If we magnify blessings as much as we magnify disappointments, we would all be much happier." ~ John Wooden

There's Always Something to Be Thankful For

There's Always Something to Be Thankful For

Manufactured by Amazon.ca
Bolton, ON